STRUCK DOWN BY AUTO-IMMUNE DISEASE

HOW I WAS FORCED TO FIND MY OWN CURE

NORMA EDMOND JOHNSON, PH.D.

STRUCK DOWN BY AUTO-IMMUNE DISEASE
HOW I WAS FORCED TO FIND MY OWN CURE

Norma Edmond Johnson, Ph.D.

MILLIGAN BOOKS   CALIFORNIA

DEDICATION

TO MY PARENTS—Regizer Bell Fields Edmond and Damon Edmond for bringing me into this beautiful world, I am eternally grateful.

To all the suffering people in this world...recognizing that there is a cure through alternative medication, without lifelong bondage to prescription drugs.

TABLE OF CONTENTS

ACKNOWLEDGMENTS

I AM A GREAT BELIEVER that we live lessons, and if we benefit from them, then we are on the right track. This book is my experience; without it, I would not have a story to tell. Shelita C. Allen, my daughter, came to my aid and helped me with the computer. without her expertise, this book wouldn't be possible.

ABOUT THE AUTHOR

NORMA EDMOND JOHNSON, PH.D., IS a resident of Inglewood, California. She is a retired teacher. She has worked fourteen years for the Los Angeles Community College Trade Technical Development Center located in Los Angeles, California. She enjoyed teaching young children and felt that caring for, loving and meeting the needs of children was her mission in life.

Norma earned a Bachelor of Arts Degree in Child Development from the University of California, Los Angeles. She holds a Master's Degree and Doctorate from Golden State University in Human Development. Dr. Johnson is a certified drug and alcohol counselor and a certified yoga instructor.

Dr. Johnson wrote a handbook for training student workers. This handbook has been used by many child development centers and teachers throughout the community college district.

Dr. Johnson is currently working as a substitute teacher and a personal yoga trainer. Her mission is to show those who are not well and tired of being sick how to get well and stay well.

PREFACE

TODAY, AT THE beginning of the 21st century, America faces one of the greatest challenges of her two hundred-year history—assuring quality healthcare for all her citizens. At the birth of our nation, one of our greatest Presidents, Thomas Jefferson, began the Declaration of Independence by stating that "life, liberty, and the pursuit of happiness" are the God-given rights of every citizen.

It is significant that he put "life" first because without a healthy life, the other two cannot be achieved.

Health—not in the sense of the absence of illness, but in the broader sense of the fulfillment of our whole physical, mental, and spiritual being—is the greatest good we can know. It is necessary for achieving almost all other goods that are commonly regarded as most important in life.

It is well-known that wealth and fame bring little enjoyment if a person is ill. There is an old saying that "Health is our greatest treasure." Yet, it is a treasure most of us seldom think about until it is threatened, or we have lost it.

We live our lives day-to-day, year-to-year, engaged in an unsound lifestyle, including a lack of exercise, insufficient rest, and excessive stress, without giving a thought to how our habits may be devastating to our health. Recently this has changed. The change has come about because labor-saving devices and city living have caused many of us to adopt unnatural lifestyles that depend on processed foods, sedentary occupations, and the stress of living in overcrowded, polluted cities.

Our growing population has put ever increasing demands on our health-care system. Forty million Americans now need health insurance (nine million of these are children). Further, seventy-five million Baby Boomers will be added to our Medicare system over the next two decades. This will create a load which our existing health-care system cannot adequately handle.

Already, most of us are experiencing more difficulty and longer waits to get medical appointments. We know the difficulty of finding a doctor who will sit down and take time to listen to an explanation of our health problems and a description of the symptoms we are experiencing. Often, when we do finally get an appointment, we are given only a few minutes before being rushed out of the office, with nothing to show for our visit but a prescription.

If we are lucky and have some common and simple complaint (such as a cold), the prescription may give us temporary relief, but time and nature will provide the actual cure. As the old saying goes, "If you take everything the doctor recommends, your cold will last about seven days. If you do nothing, it will last about a week."

At other times, however, more serious illnesses occur, which time and nature alone cannot cure. In many cases, symptoms are not eased, even when we try a succession of medications given by our family doctors or specialists to whom they refer us. This is especially likely if we have been following an unhealthy lifestyle for years. Often in such cases, the diagnosis may even elude our doctor.

After we consume useless medications without success, and we've undergone a variety of tests without resulting in a diagnosis, we find ourselves caught in a situation that seems to have no exit, with an illness or illnesses that appear to have no cure.

Symptoms are relieved, only to return. New ones often take their place. Our daily lives become a nightmare of shuttling from one physician to another, trying to keep up with complicated regimens of treatments and medications. Our nightmare goes on as symptoms constantly change and reoccur. Finally the medical experts tell us our illness is chronic and incurable. The best we can expect is to remain dependent on them for symptom relief and "learn to live with it."

This is what happened to me, and this is my story. It is the story of one woman's search to regain her most important asset in life, an asset whose importance she once failed to recognize. After a succession of tests, I was told that I had not one, but three separate auto-immune diseases, lupus, scleroderma, and Raynaud's diseases, and that my illnesses were incurable!

I decided to tell my story because I believe it contains a message of hope for thousands of others who, like me, have been told they suffer from chronic and incurable illnesses.

I have met and talked to some of these people while waiting in doctors' offices. We all agree that there must be some other kind of treatment somewhere.

I am telling my story, because I know from personal experience that doctors often give up on patients after giving them negative news about their illness. And while the incurable factor may be true at our present stage of knowledge, too often that label is given too soon and too easily. It is given, not because all treatments have been exhausted, but because of doctors' one-sided education and experience which do not allow them to educate and motivate the patient to make use of what is available. They fail to recognize resources which can promote self-healing.

This is especially true of those illnesses which are not caused by a specific disease germ or the failure of a par-ticular organ, but are the result of a systemic failure of the whole body, often as a result of years of improper living. Such illness is called *systemic illness* and can be successfully dealt with by using the method I chose. The patient should be included as a part of the treatment team; his/her physical, mental, and spiritual factors must be addressed.

My purpose in writing this book is to share my personal quest for the cure of one of the most widespread and common illnesses of our time, illness of the whole person. Although it is widespread and common, it is seldom recog-nized or treated successfully by medical specialists. Rather, they focus their treatment efforts on its symptoms, which may appear in any organ or system of the body, and usually becomes chronic. This is because treatment is generally directed at symptoms rather than at their under-lying causes.

The manifestations of whole body illnesses go by names such as "auto-immune," "degenerative," etc. Because they become chronic and do not respond to symptomatic treat-ment, they are typically labeled "incurable."

In fact, they can often be successfully treated, but only by the doctor and patient working as a team. Further, this cooperative effort must be one which embraces every level of the patient's existence— physical, mental, and spiritual.

In the chapters that follow, I explain why I became ill and what led to my discovery of the cure. In the process of curing my whole body, I not only cured the symptoms which led to my search, but the treatment of other health problems I had, some dating back years.

This, then, is the story of how, in searching for a cure for three illnesses my doctors had diagnosed and pronounced incurable, I discovered a more general cure for whole body illness. In my discovery, I found the key to not merely ridding myself of the symptoms of three illnesses (lupus, scleroderma, and Raynaud's disease), but I also found the key to achieving and maintaining stable and total health.

Because the treatment program I discovered promotes total, holistic health, I now know it offers not just an answer to the problem of auto-immune disorders. It can also be an answer for thousands who suffer from other forms of chronic and unresponsive illnesses.

Therefore, I dedicate this book to all who, like me, have suffered long, searched in vain, and are still waiting for a cure. To them, my message is one of hope. *There is a cure.*

INTRODUCTION

The Author's Journey

THIS IS THE story of my illness. Having to relive my experiences in order to write has been quite a task, a lot of hard work. I have learned much from reliving all the suffering that I underwent. There are times when it all comes back too vividly.

My name is Norma Edmond Johnson; I am a retired teacher, who worked fourteen years at Los Angeles Community College Trade Technical Child Development Center. I enjoyed teaching young children. They were my mission in life. I felt I could relate to them at this critical stage in their young life, where their needs center on love, care, and understanding. But, I became ill. I truly believe that there are others like me who want to get well. But you need to understand that the cure does not always come in pill form. There is no "prescription" involved in getting well.

This book can be a tremendous help to those who are willing to take the time and effort to climb back onto the path of health and wholeness again. The method I used has helped me in *many* areas of my life.

This book is a good reference for use with various ailments. People that have tried a "quick fix" and found that it did not work should use this method to regain their health.

I was born in Slidell, Louisiana, the eighth of nine children. My parents did not talk much to us. I learned through words and deeds. Later in life, I learned how other children are treated growing up. That's when I knew I did not like my childhood. Unfortunately, my father died when I was very young; my mother was left to care for us three girls and my one brother living at home. He played the father role in many instances.

I was very thankful when we moved into town because life was hard, living on our farm. We children had many daily chores. My parents were more interested in what we needed to do around the house than what our schoolwork was all about.

I liked being with my family, especially my sisters. We saw each other daily at school. When my sisters dropped out of school, I was very sad. I wanted to drop out, too, but I did not. I was just unhappy. I felt alone with no one to talk to, no one to share my day with.

After my father passed away, we moved around to a couple of cities in Louisiana and then to California. I adapted to moving over time. I worked at night at a soda fountain when I was in high school. Graduating from high school was a special and happy occasion for me, because I was the only child in my family to get past the third grade.

Within a year after graduation, I was briefly married to a wonderful man. We had one lovely daughter. Tragically, my husband was killed in an automobile accident early in our marriage. I was angry with my husband, because I was left alone with a child to care for. But, with time, I got used to being alone again. However, I knew that I was not really alone. I had my daughter and my "higher power," and that was all I needed.

I worked at a factory for a long time. Then I worked at Los Angeles Unified School District, where I was employed as an educational aide and teacher for many years. I learned a great deal from my colleagues about children. In time, I learned some unhealthy behavior, too, as I began to drink alcohol and smoke cigarettes. This behavior became part of my life for many years.

As my daughter was growing up, I wanted many wonderful things for her. I realized that the only way to make a better life for us was for me to return to school and get a better education. I was excited about my decision. My head was on straighter than I thought!

My education began at California State University, Los Angeles, where I earned a Bachelor of Arts in Child Development. I attended night classes and worked eight-hour days. At the University of California, Los Angeles, I received a certification for counseling in drugs and alcohol. Later, I became a certified yoga instructor. Eventually I earned a Master's and Doctorate from Golden State University in Human Development. I loved God so much, I felt the need to know more about Him, so I received an ordination from Community Church by the Bay, under Dr. W. Parker, Newport Beach, California.

While teaching at Trade Technical College, I wrote the handbook on training student workers. Teachers at nine child development centers throughout the community college district used this handbook.

Looking over my life, I discovered I had many talents and felt so blessed. I thanked God for making it all possible. One talent I developed was writing. I had thought of writing a book when I retired, but I never thought it would be about my health.

I was at the peak of my career with many accomplishments when disaster struck. I knew I was not taking care of myself, especially in the area of nutrition. I had developed poor eating habits because of the pressures revolving around my studies while I was in school.

I went to a nutritionist, and that was when I learned how unhealthy my diet was. I found out that sooner or later, your body will let you down when you fail to treat it right. The immune system stops functioning properly, allowing the body to become vulnerable to toxins and germs. I knew that my eating habits were not conducive to healthy living, but somehow, I thought that everything would be all right. Well, I'm here to tell you that it does *not* work that way. My nutritionist and I talked for hours. She introduced me to a healthy way of eating and taught me the importance of eating healthy foods. She also introduced me to yoga classes, where I learned more about eating healthy. The education I received from the nutritionist helped me enormously through the next three years, and it still remains part of my daily regimen of healthful living.

It was not until some years later that I discovered I had scleroderma. That knowledge was my first step in the right direction. The disease made me feel as if my body were being attacked and hugged too tightly all over. I was aware that something was happening to my mind and body. I was in shock and did not know what to do.

Then, lurking in the background and waiting for the right moment to further pounce on my already weakened body was lupus. Lupus is a disease that gives you a terrible feeling all over. It leaves you tired, with no energy, easy prey for overwhelming depression. This depression came from the realization that I had a chronic disease, with no probable cure. Since my mind was numb, it took a while before I could decide what to do.

I knew that, somehow, I must change my attitude (and become more positive) and behavior (and develop better habits while ridding myself of the bad ones). I knew that the mind has a powerful effect on health. Changing my outlook would not be easy.

I was still working forty hours a week and had no opportunity to give myself the care that I needed.

Care for my kind of illnesses is a full-time responsibility and could take years before I might find a cure.

Even today, knowing what I do and where I've come from, I am still bewildered about how I managed to bring it all to pass. I knew that meditation and prayer were important to the healing process. I also realized that I needed support from others that understood me and sympathized with what I was trying to do. It was hard for those close to me to understand what I was going through, because my diseases were invisible. If I had had a broken leg or were bleeding, the visibility would have made understanding and acceptance easier, but my auto-immune diseases were hidden. Some people found it difficult to believe that I was ill.

Despite disbelief on the part of others, I began to search within myself for a more positive outlook, while I began seeking help from others. My mother often said, "When you don't know what to do, stop and pray about it." My grandmother would have said, "Stop, be still, and the answer will come."

During this time, I went for a walk five or six mornings a week. It felt good out there. Occasionally, my neighbor would walk with me and always showed concern about how I felt. That encouraged me. It's a good feeling when someone gives you needed support.

My daughter called often. She would never admit that I was ill. I suppose her denial was because she was afraid my illness would hurt her well-being in some way. She always thought of me as a strong person. Perhaps if she admitted I was ill, she might feel I would not be there for her when she needed me. Or perhaps she felt I was too strong to become ill.

There were times when I felt myself getting worse, hurting in areas of my body that never hurt before, not being able to sleep at night, and uninterested in food. Depressed, I wanted to sleep all day.

Meditation was my savior. It was the place where my great ideas were born. I came to realize that my attitude had a lot to do with the way I felt about the things that were happening. I realized that I needed to spend my time more wisely, thinking about alternative methods of healing in order to make me better. Positive thinking is part of the healing process and is crucial for optional health.

The professionals that helped me are aware of many of the methods I used. But it is the *medical* professionals that need to be aware that auto-immune disease cannot be cured with merely a prescribed medication.

CHAPTER 1

⊙═‹· ⊙═‹· ⊙═‹·

From Health to Illness

I CARRIED ANGER IN MY body, well into adulthood for many years. I tried very hard to make my childhood right, but it was not possible. I had always felt that I was almost alone with my problems. I never felt wanted or loved by my parents.

My first husband passed away from an automobile accident early in our marriage. We had one daughter, and my husband was a loving father. There were two other marriages after that. They both ended in divorce. I can't say my anger caused the divorce, but I am sure it contributed to it.

After returning to school and finishing part of my education, I began teaching young children. I had started the fulfillment of my strongest dream. This, coupled with the fact that my daughter was doing well in school, made me feel turned onto life.

Diagnosis "incurable"

Later, when I was diagnosed with a disease called scleroderma, it was a shocking experience. It was as if a shadow had darkened my life. The skin on my body was so tight, I could not move without effort. My immune system was weakened throughout my body. Scleroderma affected both the inside, as well as the outside, of my body. When the outside becomes tight, much damage is being done to the inside vital organs.

When I eventually attended scleroderma meetings in the community, alternative therapy was not recommended because those present did not know much about herbs and other approaches to treatment. That's why I am writing this book, so others who suffer can understand that one size, or one therapeutic approach, does not fit all. Scleroderma effects us all differently, and that's why treatment differs from person to person. This strange effect that the disease had on me may be different for someone else.

When I discovered I had Raynaud's disease, it was a frightening experience. All of a sudden, my entire body became cold inside as well as outside.

When my body started to warm, the extremities were the last places to feel it. If any of these parts got injured, infection would set in and gangrene might become a real problem, because the blood supply becomes limited. It was imperative that I strengthen my immune system as rapidly as possible.

Then I was diagnosed with lupus, at which point I began to feel the greatest pity for myself. There was not one place on my body that did not hurt. I felt alone and helpless. This was one of the times I just had to suffer through it and try to think of something that might help me feel better. Lupus is unpredictable and attacks one organ after the other. It causes all the body organs to weaken and perform inadequately.

I think I became ill primarily because my body had carried resentment for such a long time. My thinking processes were distorted and making right decisions was impossible. I felt wounded from childhood. I had made many mistakes. Two marriages that did not work only reinforced the feeling of being unloved. There were many times I felt overwhelmed by life. I felt confused; my thinking processes went in many scattered directions. My head felt very "busy." Intelligence was fractured and nothing of quality got done. Subconsciously, I put up barriers to keep out interference. Unfortunately, I stayed in a state of dilemma, no matter how terrifying it was, until finally, I found the will to step back into reality.

When my life situations were not so favorable, eating healthy was not possible. Most of the time, I did not eat. I was overcome with guilt, so I stayed there. My pain went unnoticed, and I tried to act as if everything was in order. Sometimes the use of stimulants helped to dull the pain. I held onto all these confused ways of thinking and these destructive habits for a long time.

I only began to see hope at the end of the tunnel when I realized that the body is designed to heal itself. The word "incurable" is so frightening. It only becomes less so when we realize it simply means that a condition cannot be cured by "outer" methods, and that we must go within to be healed.

Every society throughout the ages has had methods of healing the body, mind, and spirit. Modern medicine is good at treating acute illnesses and accidents, but poor at treating the whole person. There is prescription medicine for infections, pain, and body malfunctions, and if medication fails to cure, surgery is next in line. If it is something that surgery can't fix, then radiation and/or chemotherapy is often used. With auto-immune diseases, these kinds of approaches are futile, so we must look elsewhere.

Auto-immune diseases are not caused by germs. They are caused by a failure of the immune system to distinguish between germs and the body's own tissues. We must strengthen our immune system, so that it can, once again, take up its job of attacking invaders. This important internal army is able to destroy bacteria, viruses, fungi, and cancer cells when it is working efficiently. Unfortunately, due to poor nutrition, stress, and environmental toxins, my immune system turned away from its job of defending my body and began attacking it. The first success in restoring my own immune system came when a nutritionist put me on a healing diet.

Females account for eighty percent or more of all auto-immune diseases. This is because of the effect of female hormones on the body. Stress is among the many factors that effect immune function, because it changes hormone levels. This happens especially in mid-life when there are already so many hormone changes taking place. There are other factors that also weaken the immune system, like sleep deprivation, alcohol consumption, inadequate nutrition, excessive salt and sugar, and negative attitudes toward self and others. Most of us work at least a forty-hour week with little or no recreation. Fatigue can also be a major factor in undermining the immune system.

When my auto-immune disease began, my symptoms included change in skin color (darkening), headaches and joint pain, depression, anxiety, fatigue, constipation, arthritis, insomnia, and weight loss. When the skin discoloration occurred, I realized that it was only a manifestation of more serious changes within. I tried avoiding the sunlight, but this did nothing to address the serious problem I had. During the night, I scratched my skin in my sleep, then I had to spend time the next day trying to heal the damage I had done. The headaches were aggravated by my believing I had an incurable disease, and that there might not be any cure. I dreaded the nights because then, my mind was totally occupied about the possibility of never getting well.

My joint pain started in my left knee and two index fingers. I kept using them, but each day, they presented the same problem again. Mornings I tried showering to get the swelling under control. This helped reduce the swelling, but did not remove the pain.

I believe my depression and anxiety were, in turn, consequences of my headaches. I often used sleep as an escape from my depression. Sometimes I would sleep all morning and well into the afternoon. When I awakened, I would sometimes feel better. I would have enough energy to get dressed and fix lunch. But after preparing my lunch, I was too exhausted to eat. This went on for months. I dreaded most of my life.

Another serious problem I had concerned digestion and elimination. I began taking laxatives; sometimes they worked and when they did not, I took an enema. Like most other problems, these went on for weeks and months without any permanent relief.

I did not feel hungry most of the time. I tried to eat something before going to bed. Much of the time I only consumed soup and water. Soups were easier to make than preparing individual dishes. I also found my brain was not functioning well; it took me a while to think of what to do next. Meditation and prayer were my savior. I have my mother and grandmother to thank for this wisdom. Prayer I knew, but meditation I had to learn, and it was a wonderful and rewarding experience. Sometimes I would walk while I meditated. I looked forward to walking each morning. It would take over twenty minutes to walk one mile. It felt good just to be out there.

When I took medicine, I did not feel any better; in general, I found good nutrition made me feel better than medicine. Some doctors get carried away with the belief that allergies are to blame for whatever ails you. Doctors try to substitute drugs for sound nutrition. For me, drugs were not the answer; it was *nutrition* that worked for me. Doctors' thinking seems to be, "If I can't find a drug for it, then it can't be cured." I came to believe auto-immune disease is something medicine doesn't help. Detoxification, prayer, meditation, just to name a few treatments, that do help. With these methods, there are no detrimental side effects.

From my experience, it is a waste of time to explore temporary relief from drugs or modes of treatment that are far less effective than what I discovered. First, however, we must detoxify. It takes time for drugs to get out of the system before true healing can take place.

I remember doctors lecturing me, "Take medication, and you will feel better." I took the medicine, and I did *not* feel better. The medication is experimental and designed to relieve symptoms. When I turned to other methods for healing, I really began, for the first time, to see *permanent* improvement.

I did research to learn about my diseases and learn what I could do to heal myself. From time to time, I would talk to someone who had the same problem. Just like me, they had no knowledge about the disease. I eventually found two or three lines about auto-immune disease in a magazine article and heard a little about it on television. I joined a support group. Then one day while shopping at a health food store, I saw an article on auto-immune disease, which spoke about healthy foods to eat. After that, I made monthly trips to at least four health food stores to see if they had information available. In the support group, I also found help from lectures by health-care experts. From the research I had done, I knew I was going in the right direction. I began to eat a healthy diet, exercised daily, prayed, and meditated to heal myself. I also began to address my personal, emotional, and spiritual issues. At last, I was on the road to recovery.

CHAPTER 2

Anatomy of an Illness

AUTO-IMMUNE DISEASE—WHAT IS IT?

FIRST, LET'S DEFINE WHAT AN auto-immune disease is. According to *Taber's Cyclopedia Medical Dictionary*, it is a disease produced when the body's normal tolerance of its own antigenic markers on cells disappears.

My first important discovery on the long road to a cure was that my various "diseases" were manifestations of a *single* disease. I discovered this through reading and studying myself.

Early in my illness, I detoxified my body and walked and practiced yoga daily. By eating a healthy diet and using meditation and prayer, I spent most of my day doing all positive things, as well as reading articles concerning my illnesses. Often the articles I read said the same thing. I never stopped searching for new information about the diseases. When one has suffered with pain as I did, death would have been welcomed. And no effort was too great in trying to find relief.

Another one of my trial and errors was that I mixed a variety of cleansing herbs and took them into my body twice daily for about three weeks. When I did this, I began to feel much better. Viruses and bacteria are living organisms that prey on us when our immune system is weak. Because of poor diets, stress, tobacco, and alcohol abuse, along with certain medications, the immune system becomes compromised. When we are in a run-down state, it creates the perfect environment for viruses and bacteria to infiltrate our body and flourish. At that point, our immune defenses break down, and we develop the physical symptoms of illness. The cleansing herbs were what my body needed to help restore the immune defenses and to get better. My grandmother used to say, "Nine out of every ten people could get well if they would do it God's way." I think that the labels doctors give illnesses make it difficult to understand whatever it is you need to know. When my skin began to get tight, doctors called it "scleroderma." When parts of my body turned dark and I began having problems in my internal organs, it was "lupus." When my circulatory system gave me problems, it was called "Raynaud's disease." After much research, I discovered these are all the result of a weakened immune system. I also found there are many nutrients that can be combined to reinforce and stimulate the body's defenses against this problem.

I then began to realize what was happening to my body. I had now discovered what I had done wrong in the past that weakened my immune system and what I could do right in the present to turn that around.

One of the first things I did was to get some tests done by a doctor, then I performed tests that I could do myself. The upper GI series (barium swallow), an X-ray diagnostic tool for disorders of the gastrointestinal tract, was done by the doctor. The endoscopy is another diagnostic tool that is sometimes used to take a closer look. This examination involves the esophagus, stomach, and duodenum. The colonoscopy is for diagnosing abnormalities of the colon and detecting early signs of colon and rectal cancer. These tests were all given to me, because I had experienced problems in these areas. The difficulty with these tests is that they look only at one thing or one set of things in the body and disregard the fact that these systems are all interconnected in some way.

I wanted to know how my thyroid was functioning. Thyroid function is analyzed with a sample of blood. I had been told by my chiropractor that if you don't heal the thyroid, it is difficult to heal other parts of the body. Then, finally, I had a complete stool analysis. This test is performed with a stool you collect at home and send to a laboratory. After all these tests, I learned that these symptoms were due to one cause—auto-immune disease.

In trying to find a cure, I learned how to buy and prepare nutritious food. Nutrition is highly individualized; different people have different needs. Supplements also are individualized and must be changed from time to time. As I began to alter my daily routine, I developed a new outlook on life. Changing my daily routine was a big shift for me to make. I had to forgive myself and become a more positive person. This shift not only helped my body, but also enhanced my ability to truly enjoy life. It was a lot of work, and it was all up to me. Also I needed to learn to give to other people and receive from them with ease. Once I started to move in this direction, I could see and feel the difference it made in my life. I began to gain insight into many of my psychological and emotional problems. When I began to expand as a person and began thinking less about my own problems and more about others, the pain was not so great. I also started to sleep longer during the night and not dread the mornings. I made small, meaningful changes in my life.

My massage therapist and chiropractor helped me greatly. When I no longer focused on myself, I began to see the bigger picture. The more I shared with others, the more I got outside of myself and the less preoccupied I was with my own complaints and problems. I eventually found that I was giving without thinking about how I was going to get back. That's when I knew I was well on my way towards healing. I found myself getting angry less often and giving other people the room they needed to help me become a bigger and better person, and that helped promoted my healing process. This attitude kept me more in charge of my life and reduced my stress. I kept this attitude, and I felt more in charge. Stress had always been something I was powerless to handle. I have gotten better at dealing with stress through the years. I do believe for me that psychological and emotional healing was the key to regaining my health.

Auto-immune disease is a disease that can be managed with a holistic approach. I don't think psychological and emotional healing always require digging deeply into ourselves. We simply have to recognize that there are such issues that may be at the root of our health concerns.

I had a conversation with my herbalist, in which he said, "You know, we can give you as many herbs as you have money to buy, but unless you get your head straight, the herbs alone will not help." He knew what he was talking about. I thought about our conservation time after time over the years, and it made more sense to me as time went by.

Auto-immune disease—a holistic illness

I noticed that people with auto-immune disease have similar backgrounds of unfortunate life experiences. Alma, a person I talked to many times at the meetings, was a single mother with one daughter, a girl who was very adventurous. After high school, the daughter joined the Peace Corps, and later the army. Alma constantly worried, not knowing where her ex–husband or daughter were. We talked many times, and it was always the same. Susie, a long time friend, was very unhappy in her marriage and her life; in addition, her parents were having health problems. I realized that, like me, these two people had psychological and emotional problems that underlay their health problems, and that these needed to be dealt with before they could begin the healing process. I spoke to other women who were also reluctant to face their underlying psychological and emotional problems—such as marriage and divorce—which were causing their health conditions. I began to realize we could not expect our medical doctors to deal with such problems. Solving personal problems that make us ill is *our* responsibility; we have to resolve the issues. Doctors deal with auto-immune disease on a one-size-fits-all basis. My doctor was not giving me the kind of help I needed. I knew I needed to take responsibility for fixing my own psychological and emotional wounds. In trying to deal with these problems, I turned to health-care professionals other than medical doctors. I am happy I chose the path of self-empowerment to improve my health.

Ever since my high school days, I was involved with various forms of exercise. I had attended dance class, I was active in sports like basketball and track, and I was also a cheerleader. As a young adult, I attended the local YWCA. Years later, health spas became popular. I was one of the first ones there. Yoga was a new exercise to me; it was one form of exercise I had never considered. My nutritionist suggested that I take yoga classes because they might be helpful. I fell in love with yoga. I liked this form of exercise so much that I became a certified yoga instructor and taught it for many years.

Yoga *asanas* (various yogic postures) are used to maintain a healthy mind in a healthy body; their continuing and expanding use has led to widespread use of yoga as a healing technique. During the six thousand years of its known existence, yoga has evolved as a philosophy, embracing every aspect of life: physical, emotional, mental, and spiritual. The major philosophies of yoga were developed and published in texts in India beginning 300 B.C. Yoga came to the West about a century ago with soldiers from India. Meditation was mysterious to me at first, but now it is second nature. I like the way I feel when I meditate. Sitting in a quiet place, feet flat on the floor, being aware of my breath going in and out for as long as I like, puts me in a different world where I leave all emotional and physical problems behind.

One of the most important agents of healing is detoxification of the body. My nutritional counselor suggested I start taking care of my colon with colonics at least once a month. Since my body is very sensitive to chemicals, I decided to put together some natural products for cleaning. (I put the cleaning agents I had under the sink outside until I was ready to use them.) I began to do regular body cleansing, at the same time cleaning my home environment.

With the colonics, I was now addressing my problem of immune deficiency at the psychological, emotional, and physical levels. My improvement assured me I was, at last, on the road to a cure. Everything I was doing felt right and good.

CHAPTER 3

Anatomy of Health

TRADITIONAL MEDICINE STATES THAT HEALTH is not just the absence of illness. It is also said that people who are "healthy" can have subclinical illnesses. Take, for example, high blood pressure, or hypertension, a condition in which the pressure of the blood in the arteries is too high. If it goes unchecked, it leads to a host of complications, heart attacks, and strokes. There are steps that can be taken to help prevent high blood pressure in the future. These are lifestyle changes, which help treat it without drugs. When lifestyle changes are not met, the brain and other organs malfunction. When these conditions keep happening over and over again, other parts of the body become affected.

Somehow, people must face what they fear. There once was a man "shot through the heart," so it seemed to him at the time. To him, it was safer to avoid confronting his adulterous wife with his suspicion that she was cheating on him. He had fear, hurt, and anger. This underground anger, hurt, and unrest in his body manifested into chest pains. He needed to deal with his wife and her cheating, but as so many people do, he had hoped that by not confronting the problem, it would go away. This "safe" approach cost him his health. In the case of people with high blood pressure, if they would make some lifestyle changes, such as load up on fruit and vegetables, skip or reduce salt intake, and trim down if they are overweight, the progression of the disease would cease somewhat. If people with unresolved issues choose not to confront them, the progression will never end. In order to heal, a person must change his method of operation and not let his fear get the best of him.

Living with these "subclinical" illnesses is living in the "gray area," where you are not well enough to be really healthy, yet not ill enough to be really sick. But over time and with age, the "gray area" person becomes a seriously, chronically ill person.

We need to pay attention to ourselves, our bodies, and our minds early enough in life so it will make a difference. So many of us go through life not paying attention to our own lives, therefore, we do not attend to our own needs. When I was very young, much of my life was gloomy and helpless. I did not have good role models growing up. I am not saying my parents were bad people; they knew a lot of things, and naturally, there were some things they just did not know. You can't give what you don't have. Of course, I was not aware of this until later in life. In my case, it was not knowing what to do. Most of what I know, I learned from people outside my family. Throughout my life, if someone had something I needed or wanted, I modeled myself after that person.

Keys to holistic health

When I go into a health food restaurant, I look not only at the menu. I get a good sense if the place is all right. If I notice that the owner and the cook are in conflict, or that the waiters are unhappy for any reason, I quietly leave. I do not want to ingest health food contaminated by anger. It is important to know that spiritual healing can be obtained through the blessing of food. I bless my food each and every time I sit down to eat. I generally eat at home. I grow some of my favorite fruit, vegetables, and herbs between my flowers—collard greens, parsley, rosemary, lavender, fennel, cantaloupe, white potatoes, mint, and catnip. I understand the importance of fresh natural food and eating in an environment of good vibrations. It not only makes me healthier and more powerful, but more spiritual as well. And I also understand better how developing my spiritual nature and spiritual awareness can help me eat better.

Spiritual food and natural food are a good combination with Mother Nature and Father God. I suppose I did what Adam and Eve did when they ate the wrong food. I ate the wrong foods, and I suffered the consequences. I did learn from my mistakes and repented. I have learned so much about life from being ill, I feel as if I never knew anything about life before this. Holistic health has enriched my life in so many ways. It is something that needs to be experienced. Intellectual understanding is not enough.

We do not learn to drive a car by learning all about driving a car. We must drive it. We must experience it. And even then, at first, we are puzzled; we spend a great deal of time and energy translating intellectual data and our perception into movement of the steering wheel, the pedals, and the blinkers. We are tense and anxious. But once we are familiar with the road and the vehicle through experience, rather than intellectual knowledge, or from the observation of another person driving, our driving becomes easier and easier. Then and only then do we take full responsibility for driving the vehicle. (No instructor in case of an emergency.) Then we can have peace of mind while driving. As time goes by, we can enjoy carefree driving. We drive almost automatically and feel free to think, plan, and imagine at the same time. All this time, we have stored information so if an emergency occurs, our radar flashes us to take swift and correct action. The freer and more aware you are, the more relaxed you become and the more energy you save. This is one of the secrets of holistic health.

Another key to holistic health is learning to rise above the material world. This does not mean we need to give up our material nature. But we need to know there is more to life than we are able to perceive with our five senses. This inspired me to believe in self-healing and the healing of my life problems. Meditation is one powerful and safe way to achieve this freedom. Other related areas like imagination, self-improvement, love, and relaxation help people know that they are getting in tune with the universe. At first there may be a need to go back to the beginning and let go and experience the glowing warmth of the great loving flow throughout the body.

One of the best ways to holistic health is total acceptance of life as a series of lessons. This attitude will remove much of the stress of everyday life and the painful experiences of the past or the dread of tomorrow. If we try to kill the pain with drugs and alcohol, or prayer, it will rise again. I know; I tried it. We may need greater and greater doses of painkillers, which also may be destroying our organs, and disturbing our mental and spiritual balance. The problems we had in the past are still there; we need to bring them out. Only by learning from a painful problem can we release ourselves from it.

I believe everything that happens to us is for a reason, because life is an unbroken chain of cause and effect. Even a painful experience is for a reason. And since every experience is an opportunity for learning and growth, every problem, mistake, failure, and pain is beneficial, if we are willing to learn from it. Holistic healing is not brooding over mistakes, but accepting them and learning from them. In spite of our mistakes, our self-image heightens and the flow of our love and energy increases. When we expand our awareness, our lessons are not so hard. In our everyday life and spiritual development, expanded awareness will provide us with foresight that will guide us toward the right path. When our awareness "radar" detects something ahead, we can better assess the situation. The more aware we are, the better evaluation we will make. Holistic health is the continuing presence of the best functioning of the entire person at physical, mental, and spiritual levels.

As we develop our sense of movement of life through expanded awareness, the bending and focusing of energies will become easier and easier, and our living will be transformed into a feeling of fulfillment. As we grow, we are not afraid of problems any more. By learning from difficulties, I have fewer and fewer problems. From my failures, I grow; with obstacles, I get stronger. I get stronger learning from my enemies, too. I am getting better. I feel flexible and free. I can fall and rise again. My mission in life is to grow stronger and stronger with every experience. Today, I accept life; I love and flow with life. This is the holistic lifestyle that I will have for the rest of this life. Today, I am a very confident person for having chosen this path.

I had a lesson to learn, and it had to be learned well. An incomplete lesson would cause me to repeat the past. You have to know that the disease, or at least its roots, may be stealthily harboring an attack. To heal holistically, I had to become whole; one problem cannot be healed at the expense of the other. The purpose of healing is to heal the whole person— mind, soul, and body in harmony. Some of the "gray area" symptoms are caused by: poor diet, lack of exercise, negative emotions, body toxicity, stressful living, and lack of sufficient rest.

Poor diet: "Our greatest task is to learn not to interfere with this natural and spontaneous healing force (i.e., a proper diet)." I list unnatural foods and drugs as interferences with the flow. Understanding this will immediately give us more motivation to eat naturally, and to replace drugs with healing foods, herbs, vitamins, minerals, and other natural food supplements. The value of eating correctly will be further enhanced when we become aware of the vital life force that can be received through health foods.

Lack of exercise: I love exercising. Exercise reduces stress and elevates mood. Both of these aspects have a positive affect on the immune system. Allow me to share with you the four basic principles of exercise.

- *Posture:* As we age, our daily activities, gravity, and musculoskeletal changes can all contribute to poor posture. Unless we correct our posture throughout the day, the shoulders become rounded, the head moves forward, and the spine tends to curve forward. In our daily lives, we carry out so many activities in front of our bodies, that the chest and shoulder muscles become shortened and strong, while our back muscles become stretched out and weak.

- *Balance:* Our muscles work as a team. The biceps are stronger and overpower our triceps. It is important to include special tricep-strengthening exercises to keep the muscles in balance with each other. Focus on strengthening weak muscles and stretching tight, shortened ones.

- *Breathing:* If posture is poor, breathing is less efficient because there's not much room to expand the lungs. Since most of the blood vessels are in the lower part of the lungs, we must breathe deeply to pull oxygen into our lungs.

- *Brain:* Our brain could use some "muscle-flexing." We need to expose ourselves to new material, learn and use new words, practice listening, practice some form of arithmetic. The body and brain benefit from physical exercise.

Negative emotions: These emotions can be overcome from within. The real work is up to you. Take small steps toward inner change; it worked for me, and I know it will work for you.

My changes began when I started being more proactive. I tried very hard not to react to situations that bothered me. I also became more compassionate toward others. I started a block club. In the mornings while watering the grass, I made it my responsibility to keep a watchful eye open for certain children on their way to school. These children were alone most of the time. I started to feel more positive and healthy about my life. By giving to others, I felt larger. We humans are interconnected with each other, and we cannot truly be well unless we nurture those connections. Learning to be a more giving person made me a more proactive person who takes the lead in establishing and contributing to a more caring world for everyone. To me, this is like taking a holistic pill that satisfies our greatest emotional and psychological needs. Visualize total health when you give to others

and when you share your thoughts, fears, and vulner-
abilities with them. When we begin to see that we
are more proactive and more sensitive to the needs
of others, our stress, worry, fear, anxiety, and depression receive small doses of remission. Let's supply
this to ourselves and create the greatest sense of con-
tentment and well-being.

Toxins are carried in our bodies and should be
eliminated. Toxins deposit themselves in tissue and
cause distress on muscles and joints, especially in the
head and neck. They are always on the move to some
system of the body. Some methods I used to eliminate toxins were exercise, fasting, and massage. When
I changed my diet, I was eliminating the toxins I was
putting in my body. I cut down on mucus-forming
foods and instead of drugs, I used herbs and vitamins.

Stress & rest: When we become more relaxed,
when we breathe deeply, we handle stress better, and
we tend to relax more. Everything gets better when
we have more control over our lives. One of the important keys to healing is rest.

To overcome auto-immune disease, I needed to
get to optimal health. I corrected all the gray areas of
my body. Meditation, which slows the heartbeat,
eases muscle tension, and lowers blood pressure, is
therapy for stress-related diseases such as an auto-
immune disease. This is only a partial list of the many
benefits of meditation. The acupuncturist says that
disease results when the flow of energy along the
meridians is blocked; for a healthy state, the *ch'i* must
flow unobstructed along the meridians. Locating the
obstruction and stimulating or relaxing that point with

acupuncture makes the pain and/or disease disappear, as the balance of energy is restored.

Colonics are glorified enemas using many gallons of water, but only a pint or two at a time. They are given by a colonic operator, with the water flow and expulsion under the control of the operator, while the patient lies relaxed on an appropriate table, which is connected to the colonic equipment. To be efficient, colon irrigation requires a period of half an hour; during that time, 20 to 30 gallons of water may have been inserted into the colon through the rectum at the rate of only one pint to perhaps two quarts of water at a time, and then expelled each time.

Proper nutrition, cleanliness, adequate rest and recreation, regular exercise, and a positive outlook on life put these keys to good health on your ring of power. Keep the doors to immune responses open. If any one of these is missing, chances are that good health is elusive.

CHAPTER 4

Optimum Nutrition

As I STATED EARLIER, A nutritionist was the first health-care professional I contacted. She gave me a nutritional plan based on my unique needs. It was a great learning experience for me, a discovery of a whole new way of taking charge of my health. The nutritionist spent many hours teaching me information I needed for a healthy life. We went shopping at health food stores. She came to my house, looked through my kitchen cupboards, and gave me my initial lesson in organizing this new knowledge. She suggested I practice yoga since it might be beneficial to me. My other health-care professionals agreed with her. I began reading more about nutrition and recalling my nutrition classes from college.

At the support groups on auto-immune disease, I talked to some of the other ladies and told them about the first step I had taken. One lady replied, "I don't know when I'm going to die. I plan to enjoy the rest of my days." Another lady said, "I have to have something to eat (that I enjoy) before I take my medicine."

I was surprised at the fact that they both bought into the idea that there is no cure, and that they were willing to live with whatever their illnesses brought them, without seeking alternative methods of countering these illnesses.

Basic diet

When I became ill, I knew how to put a meal together and be well fed. I had learned sufficient information from my health-care professionals and felt confident enough to take charge of this area of my life. I read many books on nutrition and health and am very thankful for the background I have on nutrition. First, I needed to ask myself questions before I got started, like, *Does my heart hurt? Why am I so anxious? I don't see as well as I used to. Am I starting to have problems with my eyes? I feel like a gray cloud is over me, and I have not had a good laugh for a long time.*

For my heart, I needed to increase my intake of fiber and folic acid. These are important nutrients for health problems. For my nervousness, I needed to increase the amount of fat I consumed, as well as my intake of vitamin B6. For my eyes, I needed more vitamin A and B2. Nutrition needs vary from person to person.

Meat, fish, poultry, dairy products, and eggs are proteins and have reasonable amounts of all the essential amino acids, plus other nutrients. They also come with large amounts of deadly saturated fats.

The richest sources of vegetable protein are legumes, dried peas, beans, lentils, black-eyed peas, chickpeas, kidney beans, pinto beans, and black beans. This protein is every bit as good as protein from fatty meat and dairy sources. Vegetarians can live on vegetable protein without ever eating a cheeseburger or tuna fish. I suggest no red meat, no pork, no fried foods, and a diet low in nuts and high-fat vegetables, along with avocados. Tofu, or soybean curd, is a white substance found in the vegetable section at the supermarket. It can be stir-fried with vegetables or combined with greens and vegetables or a salad.

To remain healthy, reduce your intake of health-damaging, highly refined sugars. Natural sugars should take up the smallest number of calories in your diet, only 10 percent or less, if refined. The best source of sugar is fruit, and that should be kept down to 10 percent. This means, two to three pieces of fruit per day. Use milk products made with skimmed or partially skimmed milk, buttermilk, or plain yogurt. Avoid the dastardly "sweet nothings." They are the sugary desserts, cookies, pastries, candy, and ice cream and should only be used once in a great while, if ever.

Fiber

Fiber performs its most essential service in one area of our bodies—our intestinal tracts. It also helps keep blood vessels and lymph channels clear and open. Its job is to keep our digestive systems running smoothly and to eliminate waste regularly. Fiber is nature's own laxative. It works by making our stools absorb more water. That increases its size and makes passing the waste easier.

We need an understanding of which foods are rich in needed nutrients, and what symptoms appear when those nutrients are deficient or absent. This may help us in the task of selecting the whole and natural foods that we need. Once the vegetable and fruit becomes juice, there is no fiber in it. Soluble fiber acts as an intestinal broom. Even though such fiber reaches the colon in microscopic particles, after traveling through the stomach, the duodenum, and finally, the twenty feet of small intestines, the colon still treats fiber particles as roughage and uses them as such. Without fiber as roughage, the colon and the body, as a whole, cannot maintain a healthy condition. When juicing, fiber can be put back into the juice. When fasting, vegetable juice is the drink of choice.

Nutraceuticals

The Recommended Daily Allowances (RDA) set by the Food and Nutrition Board of the U.S. National Academy of Science, National Research Council specify for adult males thirty-three nutrients needed for preventing overt manifestations of deficiency disease in most people. The list includes four macro-nutrients: water, carbohydrates, fats, and proteins. For vitamins, their recommendations are often inadequate for the best health. This reflects thinking of over forty years ago. The RDA states that the daily intake of vitamins for adults should be 60mg of vitamin C,

10IU vitamin E, 5000IU vitamin A, just to name a few. Recognize that the RDA is based on averages. People require individualized adjustments of these averages. We also need considerably more amounts for therapeutic recovery from illness.

Linus Pauling, PH.D., winner of two Nobel prizes, has observed that high doses of vitamins are the key to good health and long life. Pauling was a nutritionist and made his voice heard. He said, "Nutrition is individualized. Nutrition provides for our needs. Nobody knows all the facts, and nobody knows what tomorrow's breakthrough will bring, because nutrition is an ever-expanding field." According to Pauling, doctors don't know enough about the field to be conclusive, but people can find nutrition sanity by individual research and turning to a nutritionist for help.

Dr. Pauling continued, "The most important thing is the immune system. By keeping that system operating as effectively as possible, we can make a significant contribution to our own good health." Some of the vitamins required for good immunity are vitamin A, vitamin B-12, pantothenic acid, folic acid, and vitamin C. These are also the vitamins that seem to strengthen the immune system when they are taken in amounts larger than those usually recommended. These supplements are necessary for optimal health. A supplement program should also include the following:

- *Selenium,* an antioxidant, is essential to the production of a powerful enzyme called glutathione, which prevents cell damage. Selenium is one of the most potent free radical scavengers that we call antioxidants. Another study involving rheumatoid arthritis showed that selenium supplements are important in reducing the production of inflammatory prostaglandins and leukotrienes, as well as free radicals. This nutrient is important in conditions such as HIV and auto-immune disorders; it helps keep the immune system in balance.

- *COQ10* is called the miracle nutrient and is often referred to as the spark of life. By the time we are 50 years old, our COQ10 level is half what it was at 20. Scientists believe that low levels of coenzyme Q10 are directly related to an increase in heart damage, since the heart muscle is rich in CoQ10. CoQ10 should be supplemented in capsule form, as it is difficult to obtain an immune-enhancing level from the food we eat.

- *Bioflavonaids* strengthen fragile capillaries and prevent "little strokes" that lead to major ones. This substance is often found in nature, along with vitamin C.

- *Vitamin C* (ascorbic acid) is an antioxidant used for maintenance of blood vessels, healing of wounds, immune function, and iron utilization. It needs to be part of your daily regimen. No other vitamin has received as much attention as vitamin C. One study proved that it provides protection against viral infections by strengthening connective tissue. Researchers believe that it is effective in treating malignant tumors and in preventing or delaying infections. To determine your personal ascorbate requirement, start taking gram doses of vitamin C until your bowels become loose, then cut back until your bowel movements are normal. This is your personal ascorbate requirement, but it may fluctuate.

Minerals

Minerals are mighty in their ability to stave off disease. We learn more about them through the latest research. Minerals, like vitamins, are micronutrients; we need them in small amounts. But unlike vitamins, these substances come from nonliving, naturally occurring elements.

- *Calcium* helps nerves conduct impulses and protects against colorectal cancer. It also helps prevent the development of colon cancer and is essential for the manufacture of DNA coding in the cells. Of all the minerals in the body, calcium is the most abundant. The deposition of calcium in the bones is a structural process. It is almost as though the bones stretch up against the pull of gravity, raising us from the earth's surface. Without gravity, the bones begin to lose calcium. Calcium requirements can vary markedly from one individual to another. Most of it is located in the bones and teeth, about 1 percent of which is essential for the contraction of muscles.

- *Magnesium* is essential for many body functions. Deficiencies are common and result in heart attacks, kidney stones, cancer, premenstrual syndrome, and insomnia. Magnesium lowers blood pressure, prevents diabetes, keeps bones strong, and extends life. When under stress, your body requires a higher dose.

- *Iodine* is found mainly in the thyroid gland. It is an important component of the thyroid hormones essential for many body functions. Since our thyroid also controls our metabolism, a lack of this micronutrient may cause weight gain, loss of energy, and depression. Kelp is a natural source of iodine. Years ago, scientists discovered a connection between low iodine and goiter. Some believe that the body's nutritional needs should be met by seaweed and kelp as natural food sources.

The optimum diet is a raw food diet, but not everyone can immediately adopt such a diet. Some won't want it, even though it would be better for their health. I wish more would follow it. Why not take advantage of your health potential? There may be certain foods you eat raw, so you should make every effort to eat more of them. Try the farmers' market in your neighborhood. Their produce is grown without chemicals and is preferable to those with additives and pesticides. Don't be discouraged or give up if you can't obtain a 100 percent optimum diet at first. You will be healthier (and happier) if you eat raw or lightly steamed vegetables and fruits. Eliminate packaged and canned food because it is adulterated food with low nutritional value since it is processed.

Herbs

The following herbs can help you stay healthy by strengthening your immune system, as they detoxify your body. Make a tea of them anytime, day or night.

- *Ginseng* helps relieve fatigue and stress by stimulating the central nervous system and by enhancing adrenal function and overall resistance to disease.

- *Astragalus* supports every phase of immune system activity, specifically by preventing and treating respiratory infections. This herb is used to strengthen the lungs and build immune resistance to colds and flu. It is also helpful in poor digestion, low appetite, exhaustion, diarrhea, and shortness of breath.

- *Echinacea* works in two main ways. It builds up the immune system by stimulating it to build more immune cells and immune chemicals. It also stimulates these immune cells into action and heightens activity levels. These actions will help you combat any infection or disease more effectively and protect you from future invasion and illness.

- *Senna* is one of the most reliable laxatives known. It increases the intestinal peristaltic movement. *Cascara sagrada* is a bark that stimulates the secretions of the entire digestive system, including the liver, gallbladder, stomach, and pancreas. It is one of the safest tonic-laxative herbs known and can be used in moderation on a daily basis without becoming habit-forming.

- *Peppermint* exerts an anesthetic effect on the stomach's mucous membranes.

- *Cat's Claw* reduces gastrointestinal tract inflammation.

Superfoods

Wheatgrass can be purchased at health food stores. Use it therapeutically or as a supplement to your diet. It can be finely chopped and added to a salad. Take two tablespoons of wheatgrass juice, followed by six ounces of water.

Green drink is another item that is high in nutrients and is made with many green vegetables. This drink is a must for your diet.

Spirulina is a kind of algae best known for health-promoting abilities. There are two species of blue-green algae called spirulina maxima and spirulina platensis. Spirulina's unique combination of nutrients has been shown to be effective in fighting free radicals and viruses, lowering cholesterol, supporting the immune system, and inhibiting tumor growth.

Food combining

Food combining is important for proper nutrition. Digestion is not just a chemical or physical process. When food enters the body, it undergoes several changes before it is broken down. Food cannot be assimilated by the system and used by various organs unless it has first been digested and then absorbed in the digestive system. Some people feel that the combinations in which foods are eaten are important. Individuals must determine what food combinations are best for them. Not only does this vary from person to person, but as time passes, bodies require change. The most important rule for combining foods is to avoid mixing protein and carbohydrates.

The best balanced diet is usually 15 percent fat, 20 percent protein, and 65 percent complex carbohydrates. To reduce undesirable fat, use olive oil in the preparation of food. There are salt substitutes at health food stores such as tamari and Bragg's amino acids. For a sugar substitute, use dried fruit puree or honey.

My own herbal mixture

This mixture is what started the healing process for me; after taking them, I started to feel better within

four weeks. I felt as if I were healed, but I knew there
was more to come. Here are some of the herbs and
their properties which were part of my intake.

- *Oregon Grape* is useful to stimulate the secre-
  tion of bile and aid in digestion. It has a strong
  effect on the liver and has a stimulating action
  on the thyroid. It is a tonic for all the glands
  and aids in the assimilation of nutrients. Oregon grape has been used in the treatment of
  bronchial congestion.

- *Uva Ursi* is used for the treatment of bladder
  and kidney infections, hemorrhoids, as well as
  spleen, liver, and pancreas problems. Tincture
  of uva ursi was routinely prescribed in many
  European hospitals as a postpartum remedy
  to reduce hemorrhaging and restore the womb
  to normal size.

- *Burdock* provides an abundance of iron and
  promotes kidney function. It is also used in
  the treatment of arthritis, rheumatism, sciatica,
  and lumbago. The Chinese use burdock to
  eliminate excess nervous energy and also consider it to be a strengthening aphrodisiac.
  Burdock is an excellent remedy for many skin
  diseases. It also helps to cleanse the entire body.

- *Blue Flag* is a remedy for infections. Blue Flag
  formulas are excellent as a deep-acting immune
  system builder. For colds and flu, it increases
  urination and bile production and has a mild

laxative effect. It helps heal acute swelling of the tonsils and lymph nodes in the neck and jaws. It increases skin secretions, which is beneficial when using the sauna, or just sweating. Blue Flag relieves pain in the liver and gall bladder, which may occur after excessive indigestion of fatty foods. This combination of cleansing actions makes it a useful herb for chronic skin problems and constipation. In small doses, it relieves nausea and vomiting.

- *Buckthorne* is an effective remedy for constipation and regulates the bowels. It is also effective for rheumatism, gout, dropsy, and skin diseases. It produces perspiration when taken hot. It can be used externally as a wash and has a tendency to expel worms and to remove warts.

- *Bloodroot* is an excellent agency in adenoids, nasal polyps, and sore throats. The bloodroot tincture is a remedy for ringworm.

- *Red Clover* is a source of many valuable nutrients including calcium, chromium, magnesium, niacin, phosphorus, potassium, and thiamine. Red Clover is also considered to be one of the richest sources of isoflavon, a water-soluble chemical that acts like estrogen and is found in many plants.

- *Mandrake* is a very powerful glandular stimulant that should be taken in small doses and with great respect for its potency. It is excellent for the treatment of chronic liver diseases, skin eruptions, bile imbalance, and obstructions in digestion and elimination.

- *Fennel* is a very valuable seed spice, combining several herbal properties. It is an antispasmodic (which prevents and relieves spasms), carminative (helps prevent gas in the intestinal tract), expectorant (removes mucus from the lungs), and stimulant (temporarily increases body functions). It can be made into a tea using one teaspoon of seeds in a cup of boiling water; steep for twenty minutes. It can be used to treat colic, cramps, gas, and mucus. The cooled tea can also be used as eyewash and can also be made into a cough syrup.

- *Calamus Root* is an invaluable remedy for hyperacidity in the stomach and intestines. It has a beneficial effect on the liver and can be used to treat most diseases of the stomach and intestines. Calamus is a useful aid to quitting smoking, because after chewing the dried root, it causes mild nausea if smoking. It will quiet the nerves and calm the body if added to bath water.

It is important that we stay healthy throughout life. Eating healthy requires simple and delicious foods. We live in an age of many diseases and many forms of ill health. For each malady that plagues modern man, there are a host of potential remedies and cures. Modern medicine offers us surgery, radiation therapy, chemotherapy, and a staggering array of pharmaceuticals. For those who would choose less orthodox routes, there are chiropractics, acupuncture, homeopathy, nutritional therapy, and a long list of alternative methods of healing. It would be worthwhile to closely examine the most basic key to our continuing good health: *the food we eat.*

CHAPTER 5

Toxins

OFTEN THE IMMUNE SYSTEM TOXICITY begins at birth. Many of the disorders related to pregnancy result from some form of blood type incompatibility between the mother and the fetus. This causes toxemia in the fetus. In the early 1900s, doctors suspected that some forms of blood type sensitizations resulted in pregnancy toxemia (poisoning of the blood that can occur in late pregnancy and cause grave illness, or even death).

There are infectious organisms that quietly take up residence in our bodies and cause no trouble. Some even help, such as bacteria that live in our intestines and help make proteins for our bodies' needs. Some infectious organisms cause symptoms whenever they enter our body and are attacked by the immune system. The greater the number of organisms, the harder it is for the body to eliminate them, and consequently, the sicker you get. It becomes a war, and the number of organisms relative to the number of immune system white blood cells becomes critical in determining the outcome. If the immune system defenses are temporarily weakened, millions of microorganisms, or germs, can quickly establish a beachhead in their war against the body. That war occurs in our bodies, to some degree, every minute of every day. The good news is that our immune system cells usually win. Sometimes a cold virus will attack the respiratory system, which then reacts by producing phlegm. Tissues swell, and sneezing, coughing, runny nose, and other discomforts appear as symptoms. Sometimes the symptoms are immediate. But often, it takes months, even years, for them to appear. These germs are in the body, draining strength from the tissues and the immune system.

It is no surprise to find that the balance of physiological forces in the body is important for health. Health is a homeostatic relationship of balance. One critical balance is between assimilation and elimination. I believe that, in many cases, a weak organ may cause the imbalance. The elimination system is less than 100 percent efficient. Attention to providing extra bulk and roughage is vital to health. Constipation can exist when bowel movements appear to be normal. This is often due to an accumulation of feces somewhere in the colon. Constipation is a common affliction underlying many ailments. A buildup of waste within the colon causes other disturbances in the body.

We live in a toxic environment. We can limit the amount of toxins we take in through air, water, and food. We can support the body's self–cleaning mechanisms. When the liver, kidneys, bowels, and lymph system are functioning well, they will eliminate toxins quickly. Dr. A. Weil, M.D., states, "The body has its own self-cleaning, self-purifying system. The best way to protect yourself from toxicity is to keep those systems in good working order." The body, for the most part, eliminates toxins, but self-cleaning systems may falter when an individual is chronically exposed to environmental pollutants. The body can't always detoxify new, foreign substances. A long-time exposure to pollution can result in metabolic and genetic changes that affect growth, health, behavior, and resistance to disease. It may also be linked to birth defects.

Environmental pollutants

Environmental pollutants include *bichloride of mercury*, other *heavy metals*, and *carbon tetrachloride*. Low-level exposure to radiation is associated with cataracts, blood vessel damage, bone marrow depletion, tissue deterioration, and tumors, along with blood cancers. Oxidation gets the blame for much of the physical degeneration connected with aging. Studies have been conducted on oxygen and its effect on the body. Oxygen works on the human system as it does on metal; it "rusts" and ages us. Oxygen combines with the fats present in cells and produces free radicals, which cause degeneration. Oxidizing chemicals are just one environmental threat.

Despite a ban by the federal government on apple *pesticides*, recent tests in the state of Washington show dangerous levels of bug killers and other agricultural chemicals on the fruit. A total of eight pesticides were found. Infants and children are most harmed. California gets most of its apples from Washington.

The health risks associated with *dumping* are significant. Areas used for illegal dumping may be accessible to people, especially children. They contain scrapped tires, mosquitoes, and stagnant water. Severe illnesses, including encephalitis and fever, have been attributed to disease-carrying mosquitoes breeding in such areas.

Ozone is an intensely irritating gas. It can damage the lungs and airways and is found at unacceptable levels in many American cities during summer months. It causes the respiratory system to become inflamed, reddened, and swollen, with coughing, burning sensations, and shortness of breath. Research on the effects of prolonged exposure to low levels of ozone has found reduction in lung function, inflammation of the lung lining, and breathing discomfort. Ozone levels rise during May through September, when temperatures are increased.

A number of recent studies have added to the evidence that children are especially vulnerable to the harmful effects of ozone. Children spend more time outdoors in the summertime, when ozone levels are highest. They also spend more time exercising, which causes them to deeply breathe in more air, bringing more pollution into the lungs. Children with asthma are susceptible to ozone. Research shows that the effect on pregnant women's exposure to ozone causes low birth weight. For most people, breathing ability diminishes over time. Even the healthy elderly are at risk from exposure to ozone and other air pollutants, which increase susceptibility to influenza, pneumonia, and other infections.

There are many health problems that can occur due to smog exposure, most of which are nearly impossible to avoid in modern society. *Smog* means 'chemical air pollution.' It is a combination of the words "smoke" and "fog." Smog levels in a particular area depend on many factors, like automobiles, manufacturing, weather conditions, and government regulations. These problems can be serious to those with preexisting health conditions, such as asthma and emphysema. Scientific studies have shown increases in the number of lung infections, lung cancer, and emphysema. When levels of smog are high, which is often mentioned in news reports, those with heart or lung conditions are at special risk. Outdoor activities should be reduced and exercise should only be done with great caution. Those who use inhalers need to carry their medication at all times.

Smog is associated with large industrial towns and high-volume road traffic. Los Angeles has been plagued by smog since the late 1940s. Other industrial pollutants produce smoke and also combine with precipitation to produce acid rain.

Radiation is another problem. Hiroshima and Nagasaki exposed millions of people to radiation, which caused mutations in the genes, birth defects, and 17 types of cancer. Other kinds of radiation exposure are found in x-rays, mammograms, and microwave ovens.

Lead is another substance that can inhibit the functions and erode the effectiveness of antioxidants, substances which destroy free radicals. Carcinogenic substances called polynuclear aromatic hydrocarbons are formed from burning wood, coal, and tobacco. The radioactive metals released by ash from coal-burning power plants settles in our bones. This substance is found in automobile exhaust and lead-based paints. It can cause impaired mental and physical development in both fetuses and young children, decreased coordination and mental abilities, and may cause high blood pressure.

Cigarette smoke prevents cilia (hair-like projections) from "sweeping" pollutants out of our lungs. Smoking also lowers immune functions. Carbon monoxide is concentrated in cigarette smoke. This chemical impairs the ability of blood to transport oxygen to the brain. Carbon monoxide poisoning can lead to headaches, dizziness, irritability, nausea, decreased mental alertness, unconsciousness, and possible death.

If you think you can escape pollution by staying inside, think again. *The pollutants found indoors are at least as dangerous as those found outdoors.* Mental and emotional problems have been linked to fumes from gas appliances and gas stoves, as well as oil, coal, insecticides, plastics, hair spray, paint, and disinfectants. Exposure to these toxins may lead to mental confusion, physical and/or mental fatigue, depression, even severe psychotic states. You may come in contact with pollutants daily. Reduce exposure to make you and your house "healthier."

Household pollutants

Avoid *particles* in fireplaces, wood stoves, kerosene heaters, and tobacco smoke. They may affect your eyes, nose, and throat, causing irritation, respiratory infections, bronchitis, and lung cancer.

Organic pollutants such as paint, paint strippers, solvents, wood preservatives, aerosol sprays, cleansers and disinfectants, moth repellents, and air fresheners, stored fuels, automotive products, and hobby supplies may all cause headaches, loss of coordination, nausea, and damage to the liver, kidneys, and central nervous system.

Pesticides include products used to kill household pests and products used on lawns and gardens. These products need to be used where it is well ventilated and care must be taken that the lawn products don't get tracked into the house.

Formaldehye insulation in the house may cause a host of problems such as fatigue, poor memory and faulty thought processes, depression, headache, flushing, dizziness, burning eyes and throat, dermatitis, bronchitis, coughs, asthma, palpitations, arthritis, severe allergic reactions, cancer, and hemorrhaging. Formaldehyde is also found in pressed wood products, hardwood, plywood, wall paneling, drapes, textiles, and glues. It is used in trailers, energy-efficient homes, carpet dry-cleaning chemicals, rug shampoo, vinyl floor tile, gases in hospital air, and commercial cleaning solutions. Individuals who are sensitive to these chemicals report feeling dopey, dizzy, and are unable to concentrate.

Asbestos toxicity is caused by deterioration of insulation and fireproofing. Effects of exposure may not be seen for many months or years. It can cause chest and abdominal cancer and lung disease. Smokers are at higher risk of developing asbestos-induced lung cancer.

Biological pollutants include wet or moist walls, ceilings, carpets, furniture, poorly maintained humidifiers, dehumidifiers, air conditioners, and household pets. A host of illnesses and diseases may occur from biological to upper respiratory irritations.

Nitrogen dioxide and *carbon monoxide* come from unvented kerosene and gas heaters, leaking chimneys and furnaces, down-drafting from wood stoves and fireplaces, gas stoves, automobile exhaust, and tobacco smoke. They can cause persistent headaches, nausea, fatigue, blurred vision, rapid heart beat, loss of muscle control, and flu-like symptoms which may clear up upon leaving the house.

Air conditioners may increase dirt, molds, and pollen, which get into the ducts in several different ways. Dust, dirt, pollen, animal dander, skin flakes, fungi, insect parts, dust mites, carpet fibers, and construction material are pulled into the duct system when the furnace or air conditioner runs. These contaminants build up inside the air ducts over time and can help make your duct system an ideal breeding ground for fungus, mold spores, mildew, and other microbes. These contaminants can affect your health and the efficiency of your heating and cooling system. Fiberglass filters do not stop small airborne irritants such as pollen, dirt, animal dander, and dust mites. Every time the furnace or air conditioner runs, these small allergens pass through the filters and build up inside the air ducts. Fungus can grow in air ducts. Most fungi release toxic compounds and people with allergies may experience symptoms such as headache, fatigue, runny nose, and congestion.

Then consider the chemicals added to our food. The majority of *food additives* have *nothing* to do with nutritional value. These additives should be avoided because they constitute health risks. Hydrogenated fats cause cardiovascular disease and obesity. Artificial food colors cause allergies, asthma, and hyperactivity. Nitrites and nitrates are substances that can develop into nitrosamines in the body and become carcinogenic. Sulfates (sulfur dioxide and metabisulfates) can cause allergic and asthmatic reactions. Sugar and sweeteners can cause obesity, dental cavities, diabetes, and hypoglycemia, as well as increased triglycerides (blood fats) or candida (yeast infections). Artificial sweeteners (aspartame and acesulfame K saccharin) can cause behavioral problems, hyperactivity, allergies, and possibly cancer. The government cautions against the use of any artificial sweetener by children and pregnant women. MSG (monosodium glutamate) can cause common allergic and behavioral reactions including headaches, dizziness, chest pains, depression, and mood swings. Preservatives (BHT, BHA, and EDTA) also cause allergic reactions, hyperactivity, and possibly cancer. BHT may be toxic to the nervous system and the liver. Artificial flavors can cause allergic or behavioral reactions.

Refined flour is low in nutrient calories and can cause carbohydrate imbalances by altering insulin production. Excessive salt can cause blood pressure increase and fluid retention. Olestra (an artificial fat) can cause diarrhea and digestive disturbances. Insofar as it is possible, give up processed foods. Changing your shopping and eating routines isn't something you can easily do overnight. The first step is to sharpen your awareness about what you're currently eating and what it is doing to you. Then you can take steps to make the changes you desire.

Polluted water

The Bush administration announced a change to the Clean Water Act that will make it easier for companies to dispose of various kinds of industrial waste materials into the nation's waterways. With the support of the Environmental Protection Agency (EPA) and the U.S. Army Corps of Engineers, the administration's new rules allow—for the first time in 25 years—industrial wastes to be dumped in streams, lakes, rivers, and wetlands. This signifies the most destructive change made in the Clean Water Act in decades.

How about the occasional oil spills? These spillages harm commercial fishing and tourism, as well as the environment. They kill fish, shellfish, and other organisms and are deadly to sea birds and marine mammals.

Chlorination in our drinking water may cause bladder cancer and colorectal cancer. Extensive research in the United States and Canada agree with these conclusions.

CHAPTER 6

⊙══⊰⊹⊱══⊹⊰══⊹

Eliminating Toxins

I STRONGLY BELIEVE PEOPLE ARE born with a weak or sluggish assimilation and elimination system. We are constipated often and this leads to other problems. The solution is to relieve the body of its waste.

Herbal laxatives

The problem with laxatives is overuse. Herbal laxatives are non-habit forming. Dr. Weil suggests using Triphala, an herbal mixture from Ayurvedic tradition. He claims that this mixture of herbs is a superior bowel regulator. Take it regularly rather than a commercial laxative. Its benefits accumulate the longer you stay on it. This is a laxative that combines senna, licorice, cinnamon, ginger, orange peel, fennel, and coriander seed.

Fiber

Fiber is essential to maintaining safe cholesterol

levels and eliminating toxins from the bowel. A good bowel movement at least once a day is essential for a healthy immune system. If this does not occur, you are constipated, and your body has to deal with too many toxins. If you follow a typical Western diet, you are not eating enough fiber. Most Americans eat only half of the twenty-five grams of fiber daily recommended by the American Cancer Society and the American Heart Association.

Fiber is found in fruits, vegetables, legumes, and whole, unprocessed grains. Unfortunately, the breads and cereals you buy at the market have been stripped of their fiber. If you are sensitive to grains or are gluten intolerant, you should avoid grains and need to obtain your fiber from other sources. Fiber is essential for the normal function of the gut. Low-fiber diets are a major cause of many illnesses, including constipation and diverticulosis.

There are two types of fiber, soluble and insoluble. Soluble fiber is found in foods such as apples, oat bran, and broccoli. Soluble fiber can lower blood cholesterol levels, which protects against heart disease. Insoluble fiber, found in foods such as celery, fresh greens, wheat bran, and legumes like kidney and pinto beans, speeds up the movement of food through the intestines. This not only prevents constipation, but it also reduces the exposure of the gut to toxins normally found in food.

Exercise

There are two types of exercises—the general ones that are good for everyone's body and the specific exercises to correct certain conditions. Everyone needs to exercise. Consider walking or joining a health spa; practice yoga. Exercise hard enough to perspire. Perspiration is another way to eliminate toxins from the body.

Bathing

Wash your hands before preparing food. Bathing (or showering) is viewed in our society as relaxation or rejuvenation. Many people choose bathtubs that circulate and bubble the water, providing therapeutic as well as emotional benefits. The main reason for bathing is to remove dirt, dead skin cells, microorganisms, and body odor. In the United States, most people bathe daily. This is not the case in many cultures. Most body odor is caused by a combination of perspiration and bacteria. The armpit, groin, and feet are the main sites from which offensive body odors originate. Different types of bacteria flourish at different body sites, which, when combined with sweat, gives each site its unique odor.

Body odor can also be caused by ingesting certain foods and spices such as garlic, cumin, or curry, that tend to linger after being eaten. The skin produces an oily substance called sebum that helps protect it from the environment. This oil traps dirt, dust, dead cells, and odor-causing substances created by the action of bacteria in perspiration. Soap helps dissolve and remove this oily debris from the skin. Since it is necessary to remove the protective sebum during bathing in order to get rid of the debris, soap may cause dry skin, irritation, or itching after bathing. Due to the chemical mature of soap, the skin's pH is more alkaline than normal for several hours. Many people use synthetic soap, which provides a more favorable pH and often includes moisturizing agents. Apply skin creams or lotions, if needed.

To be healthy, practice good hygiene and bathe with soap and water in order to eliminate toxins from the body. There are various kinds of baths, and they should be followed by a thorough massage. Baths can be cold or hot, sitz baths and sweat baths, douches, steam baths, enemas, inhalation, and sauna baths.

Massage

A massage can do for you what you can't do for yourself. Massage increases red and white blood cells, improves circulation, provides more energy, releases endorphins (the body's natural pain killers), and improves areas of strains, sprains, spasms, and scar tissue. Massage can help relieve certain common physical problems and help bring the body back to optimal functioning. With diet and exercise, massage helps restore the contour of the body by reducing fat deposits and helping muscles stay flexible. It also reduces edema, stabilizes the spine, and increases the benefits of chiropractic adjustments.

Massage can also be an important component of your health maintenance plan. It keeps the body and mind functioning optimally, improves relaxation, immune functioning, energy flow, and reduces general muscular tension and aches. Massage is effective in combating the negative effects of aging noticeable in the middle to late years of life. It helps keep body tissue and basic functions in a more youthful state. By enhancing tissue elasticity and joint flexibility, it improves blood and lymph circulation, promotes healthy, vibrant skin, improves immune functioning, relieves muscle aches and stiffness, and relieves the effects of stress.

Massage can help in certain temporary or long-term situations which cause physical and mental suffering. It is helpful for mothers during pregnancy. It is beneficial for infants, especially premature and other developmentally retarded babies. It also helps the elderly and the disabled, especially those in wheel-chairs and those with other orthopedic conditions. Massage is frequently used to enhance the beneficial effects of other types of healthcare, such as psycho-therapy, chiropractic care, post-surgical care, and physical and occupational therapy.

CHAPTER 7

❦❦❦

Detoxification Strategies

COLONIC IRRIGATIONS AND ENEMAS

COLONIC IRRIGATIONS AND ENEMAS ARE among the most common detoxification practices. The benefits of enemas and records of their use are found in Egyptian artifacts over 4000 years old. It is clear that Galen and Hippocrates both used and taught enemas as a part of their health-care systems, and they continue to be used today. Enemas have been used successfully to stimulate the immune system in infectious diseases and to treat constipation, diarrhea, dysentery, painful menstruation, depression, toxicity, colitis, diverticulitis, common migraines, tension headaches, acne, allergies, and fever. They are also used in preparation for childbirth, for internal cleansing, and in preparation for religious rites and experiences. They continue to be used against growing orthodox medical opposition.

You would think that enemas are in the same class as blood letting to balance the humors of the body, and had been abandoned because they had been found to be either dangerous, ineffective in treating disease, or been replaced by more modern, safe treatment. However, little or no sound scientific criticism of the treatment has ever been published.

In the 1800s, almost all healers were midwives and lay nurses who worked in the fields by day, and treated their neighbors using enemas and herbs. With the rise of the scientist-doctor, the natural remedies became "old fashioned." As time went by, there were better procedures. Antibiotics and sterile techniques were developed, reducing the chances of dying from infectious disease. The very nature of healthcare changed; now it's the pill-and-scalpel era. Modern science grew rapidly during this time. As it did, it required more technical education to administer new treatments. These techniques and advances changed life for ever.

In the 1900s, there was a shift in medicine. Schools needed to be accredited and the number of them was reduced. This increased the social and financial status of physicians. The midwife became the nurse, who administered colonics and enemas.

Because the medical profession began to look at medicine to cure everything, this was one of the major reasons colonics were abandoned. The doctor passed this duty down to a nurse. Hospitals began charging enormous prices to administer a colonic. It became demeaning for the professional medical personnel to give enemas, so eventually, between 1930 and 1980, the medical profession completely abandoned colonics and reduced the use of enemas in medical practice—not because they had been proven ineffective or unsafe, but purely due to social and economic reasons.

Most chiropractors followed the same path as the medical doctors and reduced administration of enemas and colonics as part of the office visit. Curing a disease, using low-cost treatment, or proving that an adjustment would help a patient, are not in the interests of the drug industry. These things do nothing for the economic machine, except perhaps remove some of the clients who were previously using their products. Curing must be economically rewarding unless there is a threat to those in the upper class that control the economy.

Researchers like to get paid and work on projects that can generate income for them. There has been no research on enemas or colonics, because there is no money in it. The therapy only uses water, along with a therapist. There are few pure scientists who approve of the treatment and who are willing to invest their time and money into such a project, with no hope of financial or social rewards for their efforts.

Fasting

Fasting is more than just the absence of food. It is a very powerful tool for healing and strengthening the body. As with any tool, it's important to understand the proper use of fasting before starting it. Don't just go on a fast indiscriminately, because you can do more harm than good. You should prepare yourself for the fast by modifying your diet. Eliminate junk food and begin eating lighter meals composed mostly of vegetables and fruit. Then try fasting for a meal or two, then for a whole day. When you feel comfortable with light eating and occasional one-day fasting per week, you are ready to fast three to five days. People who fast for the first time are often surprised to find that sticking to their diets is only half the challenge of fasting.

Although any time is appropriate for starting a fast, springtime is best. The exact time of spring warming varies from region to region, but it is a time when the climate is changing from cold to warm and nature is reawakening. Often the physical cleansing of a fast is accompanied by a mental cleansing as well. The discipline of the fast can bring out a lot of anger and negativity. The best way to deal with inner cleansing is to stand back and let it happen.

How to break the fast is important. Fasting cleanses the body. The body is very sensitive, so break the fast slowly. Lemon, water, and some steamed vegetables are best to end it. Save the nuts and hard cheeses for later. If you have been eating junk food for a long time, or abusing your body in other ways, don't expect to entirely cleanse your system overnight. Go slowly and steadily, making dietary changes. You will see gradual improvements. Once you have effectively cleansed your system, don't expect to go back to junk foods without paying a cost for it. Your body, having become accustomed to a higher grade of fuel, will not tolerate the heavy junk food you once loved.

Once a week, give your digestive system a rest. Not only does a day off from eating give your internal organs a rest, it also breaks the "food habit" so that it is easier to regulate your diet during the rest of the week.

Chelation

Chelation therapy is far safer and much cheaper than having a by-pass operation. In some cases, this treatment may obviate the need for surgery. Protection from exposure to heavy metals is important, but like most people, you have probably been exposed to these common heavy sources over a lifetime—without even knowing it. *Chelate* means 'to latch onto.' In the case of heavy metals, the chelator attaches to the metal, then carries it into the blood and kidneys, where it is excreted by way of the urine. Although chelation will also remove other minerals along with the bad guys, your chelation physician will return these good minerals to your bloodstream to ensure adequate levels. Chelation is especially important in helping to detoxify those with auto-immune system disorders so the total toxic load can be reduced, allowing the immune system to function without an extra burden.

Toxin avoidance

Alcoholic beverages, if drunk, should be done in moderation, with meals, and when consumption does not put you or others at risk. The effects of alcohol alter judgment and can lead to dependency and a great many other serious health problems. Diseases associated with alcohol are high blood pressure, strokes, heart disease, certain cancers, accidents, violence, suicides, birth defects, cirrhosis of the liver, inflammation of the pancreas, and damage to the heart and brain. The elderly, especially, are likely to mix drugs and alcohol. They also consume thirty percent of all prescription medication. The elderly are more likely to suffer medication side effects compared to a younger person, and those effects tend to be more severe with alcohol use. Alcohol used by children and adolescents involves serious health risks and other major problems.

Tobacco smoking has been recognized as a major cause of disease and death for over forty years. In the past twenty years, a growing body of evidence has shown that exposure to environmental tobacco smoke may also be a threat to health. Scientists have documented the presence of some of the toxic and carcinogenic components of environmental tobacco smoke in the hair and body fluids of nonsmokers. Smoke is an irritant. It irritates the eyes, nose, and respiratory tract. Infants and children are at risk of respiratory and middle ear infections, asthma, and leukemia. Yet, women are smoking in increasing numbers. According to a national survey, twenty to twenty-five percent of expectant mothers continue to smoke during pregnancies. Women who smoke risk heart disease, cervical cancer, and lung cancer. They create particular risk for their offspring.

Coffee is a stimulant. It can increase mental alertness and your cholesterol levels by ten percent. The acidity in caffeine tends to give people upset stomachs. Caffeine during pregnancy is not good since its effects can be transferred to the unborn child. People who drink coffee often experience withdrawal. A small group of individuals—less than five percent—regularly experience caffeine withdrawal headaches, fatigue, and drowsiness lasting no more than a day or two when they attempt to stop use.

Teas (herbal) are used in place of caffeine-containing commercial teas and other beverages. Dietary recommendations encourage the use of herbal beverages, as well as the use of herbal seasonings to flavor food as a way to cut down on the use of table salt. Herbal products have long been used as natural remedies for the treatment of various disorders and illnesses. These can be beneficial for a whole host of common conditions. Be wary of products that are sold as cure-alls. Some of the herbs sold today are safe and may have therapeutic benefits, while others may have no measurable effects. Still others may be toxic and dangerous. Over the past decade, more than thirty herbal teas have been found to contain substances that cause serious toxicities, including disorders of the liver, nervous system, and the gastrointestinal tract, as well as blood disorders. Manufacturers are not required to list potential toxicities on the label. A number of herbal teas have been shown to contain psychoative substances and can produce adverse neurological effects including hallucinations. Among these herbs are mandrakes, nutmeg, periwinkle, yohimbe, lobelia, and thorn apple (jimsonweed). In addition, guarana and maté have stimulatory effects due to the high levels of caffeine they contain. There are many herbs that are safe to use in moderation and which contain active constituents that may have important physiological benefits.

Prepackaged food—When you are at the supermarket and pick up a can, box, or any packaged food, be sure you read the label. Be aware that some ingredients are not on the label, but may be added to the food. Shopping can be a nightmare if you are concerned about the ingredients in your food, as well as the cost. Prepackaged food usually contains a lot of extra salt, sugar, and fat. If you live on packaged food, then your salt, sugar, and fat intake will be at an unhealthy level. Eat natural, unprocessed foods whenever you can.

More toxins to be concerned about

X-rays—experiments show an undeniable relationship between leukemia and cancer and excessive exposure to x-rays. Excessive exposure to radioactive material can cause immediate radiation sickness. The effects of radiation are far greater when the whole body is exposed. Radiation exposure of pregnant women may cause microcephaly and other congenital defects in the fetus. Radiation therapy can cause leukemia in adults and other cancers in children. In diagnostic x-rays of the mother's pelvis, the gonads of the unborn child receive enough radiation to cause genetic damage and occasionally causes leukemia and cancer.

One researcher stated of his experiments, *"The mysteries of radiation are deep and far from solved. They must be approached with great respect and caution. Indiscriminate use of any type of radiation is a foolish and costly practice, whose terrible effects cannot often be corrected. It is important that doctors be aware of the danger of over-exposure to x-rays and exercise great caution in prescribing their use so that the patient is x-rayed only when it is absolutely necessary. It is a blessing that it is available, but it is a mixed blessing and must be used with full consciousness of the dangers it holds. Bearing this in mind, readers are cautioned to avoid any unnecessary sources of radiation. Regardless of what you might read or be told, irradiation in any form, and in any amount, is dangerous."*

Solvents and cleaners are dangerous. Carpets will get dirty over time. They take a lot of abuse from children and pets. Like other cleaners, carpet cleaners may contain toxic ingredients, some of which are not listed on labels because they are considered "proprietary," or "trade secrets." Some carpet cleaners, especially spot removers, can be particularly dangerous because they contain chemical solvents similar to those used by dry cleaners. These chemicals dissolve dirt without soap and water and give off strong odors. There are many ingredients in carpet cleaners, including pesticides, formaldehyde, acids, disinfectants, lye (sodium hydroxide), fragrances, and others. 3M's popular Scotchguard contains all of the above and also Teflon, which is used to coat nonstick pans. The use of these chemicals is currently under investigation.

There is some speculation that there is a link between carpet cleaners and Kawasaki disease. John Travolta and Kelly Preston's son became very ill and was rushed to the hospital, where doctors diagnosed him as suffering from Kawasaki disease, a childhood immune system disease that causes the inflammation of blood vessels throughout the body. If untreated, it may affect the heart. The parents were asked to fill out a questionnaire, which contained questions about family history and family health. One of the questions asked was if the carpets in their home had been recently cleaned. Kelly had thought that cleaning the carpets religiously was the healthy thing to do for her children. During application and while drying, the chemicals in carpet cleaners evaporate and concentrate in the air, causing indoor air pollution.

These chemicals can cause asthma attacks, congestion, sneezing, coughing, fatigue, nausea, and other symptoms. Carpet shampoos usually leave a sticky residue on carpet fibers. The residue is hard to see, though it can make carpets feel rough, and it may leave an odor. Children crawl and play on carpets. They inhale these residues and get it on their hands, which often go into their mouths. Dry shampoos, powders, and foams may also linger on carpet fibers.

Another issue related to carpet cleaning is the potential for mold growth in carpets that do not dry quickly enough. Steam-cleaning carpets can thoroughly dampen the carpet and the pad underneath.

Steam-cleaning is an invitation for mold spores to sprout. Once mold begins to grow in a carpet or its pad, it's impossible to remove it adequately. When mold is not actively growing, mold particles and spores can cause health problems such as fatigue, headaches, allergy, asthma attacks, and other respiratory difficulties.

Dry-cleaners—As part of the overall strategy to reduce cancer risk to residents, the California Air Resources Board is proposing to phase out a toxic chemical used by dry cleaners. The dry cleaners are a higher cancer risk to their neighbors than an oil refinery or power plant. Dry cleaners can help reduce the health risk by switching from known cancer-causing chemicals to proven environmentally friendly alternatives. Perchloroethylen (known as "perc") is a deadly, cancer-causing chemical used in dry cleaning. The Coast Air Quality Management District states, "We recognize that most dry cleaners are small, mom-and-pop operations and many are minority-owned. We have carefully crafted our proposal to minimize the economic burden on these businesses." Perc is known to cause cancer. In addition to being a toxic air contaminant, perc is a major water pollutant in Southern California, due to improper disposal practices in the past by various industries. Because of perc's "toxic liability," some landlords will no longer lease their property to dry cleaners.

Prescription drugs—There are now natural substances available that are able to assist the immune system with its task. Orthodox medicine provides prescriptions and other pharmaceutical drugs. The

Food and Drug Administration (FDA) provides us with drugs that suppress the symptoms of the disease, but do not cure it. Surgery is usually a temporary fix, as it does little to seek out, understand, or remove the cause of the problems. It is now well documented that prescription drugs kill 100,000 or more people in America each year when they are correctly used. The danger of their interaction with other prescription drugs is also fairly well-known, and the results of such interaction can be fatal. Everyone must use his or her own judgment to ensure that they are not damaging their health further when they take prescription drugs for extended periods of time. When natural alternatives are available, try them first.

Illegal drugs—Some of the common drugs in use today are dangerous to the well-being of the user and the people around you. Fourteen- and fifteen-year-olds often know where to obtain illegal *drugs. Many know drug users.*

People understand that when money goes from the pocket of an American to buy drugs, that money could end up financing unspeakable crimes around the world. Parents, teachers, faith organizations, and youth and community groups can answer the national call to fight terrorism by preventing illegal drug use in America.

Young people with diabetes who experiment with recreational drugs are at special risk. They should seek information on how to control their condition. Speed increases the body's metabolic rate and rapidly decreases blood sugar levels. In diabetics, this can lead to a coma and, in extreme cases, death.

Allergens—The causes and effects of allergies have long been known and can be a serious health threat. Unfortunately, allergies seem to be on the increase. They are unwanted responses of the immune system, resulting in inflammation of the eyes and nose (rhinitis), lungs (asthma), and skin (eczema). It is estimated that allergies affect some 40 percent of the population at some time and that percentage is on the increase. Allergens in the house come from dust mites, microscopic insects found in our indoor environment. The bedroom is particularly vulnerable for allergy sufferers, since we spend one-third of our life in bed and a good deal of other time there, dressing and preparing for the day. We shed skin scales (a source of food to the dust mite) in our sleeping environment, where they are collected by the linen, pillows, mattress, and carpet. All these areas are ideal breeding grounds for the dust mite.

Personal hygiene—Use a toothbrush and toothpaste to remove sticky food residue from the teeth. A mouthwash cannot do this. Teeth mainly get dirty from the "food paste" that sticks to them while we eat. Flossing cleans the in between areas of the teeth. To avoid the taste of the cleansing element found in toothpaste, flavor is added as a cover-up. The most effective ingredient found in toothpaste is an abrasive, which helps remove plaque from the teeth. Health food stores carry natural brands of toothpaste.

Mouth rinses containing alcohol can be life-threatening if ingested by young children. Therapeutic mouth rinses containing more than three grams of alcohol are dangerous. Mouthwash is very attractive to children because of the bright color and taste. Symptoms of alcohol toxicity in children include decreased inhibitions, trouble standing and walking, mild euphoria, and irritability.

Antiperspirants—Using an antiperspirant may not be good because it can clog the underarm pores. All major antiperspirants use the same active ingredient, aluminum zirconium. Some articles in the press and on the Internet have warned that underarm antiperspirants or deodorants cause breast cancer. People concerned about cancer should talk to their healthcare professionals.

Hair products—When using dyes and bleaches, hot oil treatment is used, which may also help the hair stay in good condition. There are natural hair products on the market which contain negligible amounts of lead and are readily available. These types of hair-coloring products are safer for use in the home, because they contain organic dyes and bleaches that cause immediate changes in color and require neither daily nor weekly application. They are generally advertised for women, but they are also increasingly becoming available for men. Pharmacists should warn patients that hair-coloring agents formulated with lead acetate contain between 3 and 10 times more lead than the limit allowable by law for paint. Consumers who use hair-coloring cosmetics should be guided to the numerous cosmetic products currently available that do not contain lead acetate. Pharmacists should urge that hair-coloring agents containing lead acetate be removed from the stores.

Cosmetics—We all need to follow a healthy daily routine of skin care. Begin with a good exfoliant such as glycolic acid. Avoid all conditioners containing any plastics. Our skin is the largest organ of our body. Besides holding us together, it protects us from the elements and from pollution. It breathes and excretes toxins and secretes a protective layer called the acid mantle, which helps to protect our skin and keeps the pH in a mildly acidic range. Skin care products available today are too harsh for our delicate skin. They can cause its protective acid mantle to be destroyed, exposing the skin to the elements and harmful bacteria. This often starts a vicious cycle of skin blemishes, which is typically treated by scrubbing the skin vigorously with a harsh or abrasive product.

Petroleum-based ingredients and mineral oils found in some skin care products are used because they are inexpensive, but they are not good for your skin. These contain paraffin and silicon, which are known to accumulate in the liver, kidneys, and lymph nodes. Inflammation of heart tissue and heart valves may also result from their use. These ingredients build a film on the skin and block natural processes and breathing. Some of the petroleum ingredients contained in beauty products are beeswax, shea butter, and mango seed oil.

A toxic body is one of the main causes of most of our illnesses. Every effort needs to be made to detoxify the body for best results. You, the individual, need to start with detoxification in the colon. I believe it would be a waste of time and money to start any place else. Most of us need to cleanse the colon because of our previously poor dietary habits.

During and after the cleansing, keep up good nutrition with lots of vegetables and fruit. Fast at least once a week to give the digestive tract a rest from food. Remember, the colon is the first place to start, for much cleansing is needed there.

Detoxification is one of the components to getting well and keeping well. These measures will improve your quality of health and prolong it. They are not burdensome.

CHAPTER 8

Physical Fitness

PHYSICAL FITNESS IS THE ABILITY to meet the physical demands of life. IT IS beneficial at any age. The question is, *Why exercise?* And conversely, *Why not exercise?* Perhaps the real question should be, *Do you have time for sickness?* Human beings are not well suited for a life of remote control, web hopping, and sitting for hours. I am not advocating returning to a Stone Age lifestyle, but understanding our roots helps us appreciate healthy and active lifestyles. Many of us don't have to run miles or swim the English Channel, but we need to be able to climb stairs, get up from the floor, and just be able to perform the activities of daily living. More and more research is suggesting that the greatest predictor of independent living is in the strength of the legs.

Strengthening exercises

The Department of Health and Human Services suggested that a leading factor contributing to disability and death was the sedentary lifestyle. Most of us want to have a long, healthy life span. But, many of us have some type of impairment. What we do with that impairment will determine if it becomes a disability. Many of us have back disabilities that limit our capacity for exercise. Some back-care specialists recommend training the core muscles of the body, which are the trunk muscles. As these muscles get stronger, they can protect the spine from stressful movements. The primary core muscles that need to be strengthened to protect the spine are the abdominal, oblique, spinal extensors, and the trapezium muscles. When abdominal muscles and oblique muscles are weak—and they often are—they let it all hang out. Stretching these muscles is like putting on a comfortable twenty-four-hour girdle. The tummy gets tighter and trimmer, and stronger abs make for a stronger, more injury-resistant back. These are impressive payoffs for an exercise that requires no special equipment and takes only a few minutes twice a week.

To strengthen the trapezius (upper back muscle), other muscle groups are involved—the deltoids (shoulder muscles) and biceps. Toning these muscles does more than merely improve your appearance. The shoulder joints are one of the most important and most vulnerable joints in the body. Strong shoulder muscles help stabilize this joint, allowing you to lift and carry heavy objects.

Your back extensions, which are the same as spinal extensions, together with the muscles in your abdomen, serve as protective scaffolding for the spine. This is one of the most vulnerable parts of the body because it contains so many joints. There is a joint between each of the twenty-four vertebras. The stronger your back and abdominal muscles, the less likely you are to have pain and other back problems.

Muscles that play a significant role in the control of the pelvic region are the gluteus maximus, hamstrings, quadriceps, hip flexors, and hip abductors. The hip extension works your gluteus maximus, the large muscles of your buttocks, as well as your hamstrings, the muscles just below the buttocks in the back of your thighs. Any activity that uses your legs (walking, running, skiing, biking) will be more enjoyable as these muscles get stronger. You'll also find it easier to rise from the floor or from a low chair. Our legs can move diagonally, as well as forward and backward, left and right. We use this ability for many sports (tennis, basketball, hiking, and others). This multipurpose exercise enhances those moves by strengthening the quadriceps, hip abductors, hip adductors, and hip extensors. As we get older, these muscles become increasingly important for balance. This exercise strengthens the hip flexors, the muscles you use with every movement that brings your knees up towards your chest. You need these muscles for walking, climbing stairs, and getting in and out of the bathtub. To stay pain-free, work the core muscles for a well-balanced spine. The bottom line is to have better ability to control your body during all activities of life.

Remember, exercise is an investment for life. Exercises are intended to do one thing and that is, teach us how to use our muscles properly. As a result of proper exercise, blood flows better to the brain, heart, and lungs.

Even very small changes in muscle size can make a big difference in strength, especially in people who already have lost a lot of muscle. An increase in muscle that is not even visible to the eye can be all that it takes to improve the ability to do things like get up from a chair or climb stairs. To do strength exercises, you need to lift or push weights, and you need to gradually increase the amount of weight.

Muscle cells contain long strands of protein lying next to each other. When you want your muscles to move, your brain signals your nerves to stimulate them. A chemical reaction in your muscle follows, causing the long strands of protein to slide toward and over each other, shortening the length of the muscle cells. When you "make a muscle" and see your muscle bunch up and bulge, you are watching it shorten as the protein strands slide over each other. When you do muscle-building exercises on a regular basis, the bundle of protein strands inside your muscle cells grows bigger.

Do strength exercises for all major groups at least twice a week. It's not a good idea to do strength exercises of the same muscle group two days in a row. Depending on your condition, you might need to start out using as little as one or two pounds of weight or no weight at all. The tissues that bind the structure of your body together need to adapt to strength exercises. Use a minimum of weight the first week, then gradually build up the weight. Starting out with weights that are too heavy can cause injuries.

At the same time, remember that you have to gradually add a challenging amount of weight in order to benefit from strength exercises.

When doing a strength exercise, do eight to fifteen repetitions in a row. Wait briefly, then do another set of eight to fifteen of the same exercise. Take three seconds to lift or push a weight into place. Hold the position for one second, then lower the weight, trying not to drop it. Lowering it slowly is very important. It is also very important to sit or stand with your shoulders back, but not pinched, and maintain this position while you take slow, deep breaths. You can do this anytime. If you can't lift the weight eight consecutive times, it is too heavy. Reduce the amount of weight. If you can lift a weight more than fifteen times in a row, it's too light for you. Increase the amount of weight. Stretch after strength-training exercises when your muscles are warmed up. If you stretch before strength exercises, be sure to warm up your muscles first through light walking and arm pumping. Don't hold your breath. Breathe normally. Holding your breath can cause changes in blood pressure. This is especially true for people with cardiovascular disease.

If you have special problems that limit your movement, seek advice from your health-care professional. Avoid jerking movements and "locking" joints. Breathe out as you lift or push, and breathe in as you relax. Muscle soreness lasting up to a few days and slight fatigue are normal, but exhaustion, sore joints, and unpleasant muscle pulling aren't. The latter symptoms mean you are overdoing it. None of the exercises should cause pain. Although you might not notice it as it happens, most of us lose 20 percent to 40 percent of our muscle tissue as we get older. Strength exercises can partly restore this loss.

Aerobics

Aerobic exercises are activities such as walking, jogging, swimming, and raking. These exercises increase the heart rate and breathing for an extended period of time. Build up your endurance gradually, starting out with as little as five minutes of endurance activities at a time. Your goal is to work your way up to a moderate or vigorous level that increases your breathing and heart rate.

Once you reach your goal, you can divide your exercise into sessions of ten minutes at a time, as long as they add up to a total of at least thirty minutes at the end of the day. Doing less than ten minutes at a time won't give you the desired cardiovascular and respiratory benefit. These exercises can be done daily. More is not better, and everyday is best. If you can't talk while you're exercising, it's too difficult. If you can sing, it's too easy. Endurance activities should not make you breathe so hard that you can't talk. They should not cause dizziness or chest pain. Stretch after your activities when your muscles are warm.

As you get older, your body may become less likely to trigger the urge to drink when you need water. You may need water, but you may not feel thirsty. Be sure to drink fluids when you are doing any activity that makes you lose fluid through sweat. The rule of thumb is *By the time you notice you are thirsty, you are already somewhat dehydrated.* This is important year round, but especially in hot weather. If you have some health concerns, you should talk to your health-care professional.

Wear a helmet when bicycling, protective equipment when skiing, and firm shoes when walking or jogging. When you are ready to progress, build up the amount of time you spend doing aerobic activities. First, build up the difficulty of your activities, then gradually increase your time to thirty minutes over several days, weeks, or even months. Walk longer distances, then start walking up steeper hills or walking more briskly.

Physical fitness—the major effect on health

Decline in fitness is an indication of illness and/or age. There are some exercises that are difficult for an ill or disabled person. A person with hip replacements will have difficulty with lower body exercises and floor exercises. The person with cardiovascular disease can have a change in blood pressure. This person can and must exercise the time limit and do so not too vigorously. Short workouts for those with arthritis should involve reaching and stretching exercises.

Many people have witnessed the firsthand healing power of yoga. Even science has shown that it can have a positive effect on many common illnesses that strike people over the course of their lives such as heart disease, depression, breast cancer, and diabetes. The common wisdom is that yoga helps keep us healthier throughout life, and maybe even prolongs life. Yoga does offer guidance and methodology for every stage of life. It divides life into three seasons: sunrise, midday, and sunset. It can enrich people's lives with good health, happy relationships, and peace of mind.

Early in life is when we want to break bad health habits and start good ones. If you take care of your spirituality, eat a proper diet, and stay fit, it will aid you in coping with the aging process. Control your drinking, because binge drinking will get you later in life. It affects the body in many negative ways.

By the time you reach your forties, you probably understand how your genetic background may affect your health. Update your workout and nurture yourself to maintain a healthy and relaxed attitude.

Balancing your career and family responsibilities may become overwhelming. You need the support of family, community, and church. As you grow, keep evaluating your life.

For many people, sexual health, in terms of impotence or lack of libido, becomes an issue. Body changes require adaptation. Talk to your health-care professional about your concerns and keep lines of communication open with your partner.

As we approach sixty, speak to your doctor about some routine tests for cancer and to check the state of your liver and pancreas, etc. Notify your health-care professional about memory changes. My memory decline was due to the attack on my immune system. I also had cold feet and hands, sometimes a cold nose and ears. My fingers would turn blue and white and hurt from the lack of circulation. When the body gets cold, its natural response is to conserve blood for the brain and other organs by constricting vessels in the extremities. Stress also can trigger the attack. Some drugs, including beta-blockers and tobacco, can cause blood vessels to narrow, thus restricting blood flow.

Often we develop diseases such as scleroderma, rheumatoid arthritis, and lupus. Lupus is a disorder of the immune system, known as an auto-immune disease. In these diseases, the body harms its own healthy cells and tissues. Lupus can affect many parts of the body including the joints, skin, kidneys, heart, lungs, blood vessels, and brain. Although people with the disease may have different symptoms, some of the most common ones include extreme fatigue, painful or swollen joints, unexplained fever, skin rashes, and kidney problems.

Scleroderma derives from the Greek words sclerosis meaning 'hardness' and derma meaning 'skin.' *Scleroderma* literally means 'hard skin.' It is really a symptom of a group of diseases that involve the abnormal growth of connective tissues, which support the skin and internal organs. In some forms of scleroderma, hard, tight skin is the extent of this abnormal process. In other forms, the problem goes much deeper, affecting blood vessels and internal organs like the heart. Scleroderma is called both a rheumatic and a connective tissue disease. Rheumatic disease is a group of conditions involving inflammation and/or pain in the muscles, joints, or fibrous tissue. A connective tissue disease is one that affects the major substances in the skin, tendons, and bones.

I experienced these three conditions at one time, and it was extremely difficult. For winter, I bought special clothing at the nearby ski shop for walking. The clothing was designed to retain body heat. I knew I needed exercise, so I chose walking.

I had a regimen of vitamins and herbs I took daily, like vitamins C, E, A, K, D, thiamine, B1 riboflavin, B2 niacinamide, B3 pyridoxine, B6 cobalamin, B12 folacin, and pantothenic acid, along with various minerals. These supplements improved my health and prolonged my life. It was difficult at first to consume all of them, but I did and stuck with it day after day, year after year. I also drank lots of water, which is necessary when taking so many supplements. I did all of this because healing auto-immune diseases require restoration of health in many areas of the body, not just one. Nutrition and exercise are the keys to overcoming auto-immune disease.

Besides taking supplements, you must eat balanced meals daily. And maintain daily exercise, regardless of how limited it is. Also, you should rest an hour each day, in addition to having a full night's rest. Get your life in order with family, friends, and work. For meaningful extracurricular activities, I began to teach yoga and gardening. The primary responsibility for your health is *yours*.

I cannot speak too highly of exercise. I walk three miles daily, sixteen miles a week, and do some exercise at home. At first, walking a mile took me a long time. But, as I made progress, I tackled a steep hill and continued on from there. I do a lot of yoga-controlled breathing when I walk. I routinely practice my relaxation and meditation techniques.

After a few minutes of walking, the body begins to make cortisone. A lack of it causes arthritis. If a doctor prescribes it, there may be terrible side effects because it can affect the mind and soften the spine. Producing natural cortisone by exercise is a better alternative.

No one who is able to walk need live a sedentary life because the finest exercise in the world is available to you. Sometimes when I walk, I experience slight chest pains, but this occurs only in the beginning. It seems to be caused by a failure of the arteries to feed the blood fast enough to the heart due to narrowing of arteries. I keep moving and my coronary arteries open up, and the blood flows faster. Shortly after I begin the walk, I never experience these symptoms anymore. Exercise is a powerful factor to widen arteries. Exercise is of most importance to the heart, but it is also effective in maintaining the health of other body organs and glands. Like the old adage, a *chain is as weak as its weakest link.*

If any organ is sick, there is more stress on the heart. Nutrition and exercise will build a strong body again. There is so much to learn about the body and how to care for it. Just as there is a certain way to walk correctly, there is also a certain way of exercising correctly to get its full benefit and avoid injury.

As I continued my regimen, I began to get stronger. The scleroderma and lupus disappeared. Raynaud's is the only auto-immune disease I still have, and the symptoms occur now only occasionally. I am currently using biofeedback, a technique I learned in college, to deal with this. I have trained myself "to think warm." I spend a lot of time doing this, which has resulted in me having only sporadic symptoms.

I am not happy I became ill, but I am thankful people were available to assist me. I am thankful for competent health-care professionals. I am glad I took inventory when I became ill and accepted responsibility for my health. I am glad I did not waste time trying to "fix" what was wrong, and that I stuck with my regimen, no matter how long it took. I had faith in what I was doing and knew it was the right thing to do. I kept an open mind and changed my techniques, when necessary, all the while striving for a higher quality of life.

Regularity is an important word in exercising. Make an appointment with yourself. Without regularity, the progress you make in a conditioning session one day may be completely lost when the advantage is not followed up by a workout the following day. Exercise any time of the day, but just do it. I have found that regular exercise and physical activities are very important. Studies suggest that not exercising is risky behavior. It is a major cause of degenerative diseases, and it accelerates aging.

CHAPTER 9

Stress

COPING WITH STRESS

STRESS IS UNIVERSAL. WE ALL have it, and it is almost impossible to avoid. But it can be managed and controlled. Many people think stress comes from their occupation. It might be a good idea to use the power of the mind to manage stress. It is not always possible to remove yourself from a stressful situation. For example, when we go through the checkout at the supermarket, I suspect the cashier might be under a lot of stress. Where does stress come from? It comes from change. It may be a global change that reaches into every crevice of life, such as the change that occurred September 11, 2001, when terrorists crashed airplanes into the twin towers in New York City. Or it may be something more personal, like family, job problems, or difficulties in school.

It is impossible to avoid stress, because it is impossible to avoid change. Many people try avoidance through alcohol or drugs, but they end up worse off in the end. We live in an imperfect and unpredictable world, one that is always changing. Drastic life changes can occur within the space of just 12 months, like the death of a child, the death of a relationship, or a change of residence.

Drastic changes can also take place in the body. If the brain waves change, a chain of reactions take place in the body. Some people experience high blood pressure, rapid heart beat, tense muscles, cold hands and feet, anxiety, impotence, hair loss, skin disorders, and a host of other body problems. When things don't go as planned, you don't run away from the workplace. If you think the boss is giving you a hard time, you don't punch him in the nose. These are inappropriate responses. Stress causes strain on your immune system, which can lead to illnesses such as cancer or heart disease. What is the appropriate response?

It is hardly possible to pick up a newspaper or magazine or watch television without seeing or hearing some reference to stress. Just as distress can cause disease, there are good stresses that promote wellness. Stressors are not always necessarily harmful. Winning a race or election can be just as stressful as losing. We need to develop a better understanding of how to prevent disease and promote good health through reacting to stress appropriately. Good health is more than just the absence of illness and stress. It is that state of physical and emotional well-being that is supportive to the mind and body.

The effects of stress on the immune system can result in auto-immune disease (inflammation), with resulting damage from immune attacks on the body.

Lupus and rheumatoid arthritis have shown improvement in response to a lessening of stress.

Gastrointestinal problems show a strong linkage between the brain and intestines by way of hormones and nerves. Prolonged stress can irritate the large intestine, causing diarrhea, constipation, cramping, and bloating. This may result in irritable bowel syndrome, peptic ulcers, and Crohn's disease.

Stress has significant effects on the brain, particularly the memory. The victim of stress suffers loss of concentration at work and home and may become inefficient and accident-prone. In children, the physiological responses to stress can clearly inhibit learning. There may be some memory loss with age. Stress may play an even more important role than simple aging in this process.

Stress can be a factor in many physical and emotional illnesses. It might be a good idea to talk with your health-care professional if you think you have a stress-related problem. There is no single method to deal with stress. What works for one person does not necessarily work for another. Since stress can be both positive and negative, it is best dealt with on an individual basis. A healthy diet and exercise can help you deal with stressful events. Take time for re-creation. This is just as essential as paying bills or shopping for groceries. Put humor in your life. Recall positive events in your life or watch TV comedies to help harness stress. Stress is here to stay. Learn how to cope with it. Relaxation techniques, deep-breathing exercises, meditation, and massage can also lessen its harmful effects.

Coping styles

Different people cope with stress in different ways. Children raised in the same environment may cope differently. Two children reared by abusive parents may respond very differently. One may become a passive, frightened victim, and remain that way throughout life. The other child may become openly rebellious and defiant and may even leave home early. Babies are born with their unique temperaments at birth. If we tend to be frightened, shy, active, or outgoing, it is our temperaments pushing us in these directions. We may unconsciously choose one parent to model ourselves after. Some people use a variety of coping styles, depending on the situation.

Experts state that personality is a contributing factor to illness. With the amount of evidence that exists pointing to the role emotions play in the generation of or prevention of illness, we all need to examine our emotional responses. The growing amount of information has generated a new field of psychoneuroimmunology. This very long and complex word can be broken down into three parts: *psycho* ('the mind'), *neuro* ('the nervous system'), and *immunology* ('the immune system'). This exciting field of psychoneuroimmunology (PNI) deals with how the mind, nervous system, and immune system interact to support wellness or disease.

Our emotions are manifested in our personalities. The three basic personality types are Type A, Type B, and Type C. I provide a brief description of these personality types, as well as some common diseases associated with the personality type. However, these diseases are not limited to these personality types. Nor do these diseases always manifest themselves in these personality types.

The Type A personality is well-known for its contribution to coronary artery disease and heart disease. A person with this personality is quick to anger, impatient, nervous, and often stressed out. Heart disease is the number one killer in America, and this personality type is especially vulnerable. Type A individuals harbor an excessive amount of competitiveness, aggressiveness, and a sense of urgency. A free-floating anxiety is often accompanied by hostility. Type A is often associated with executive or leadership positions.

Type B personalities are at a lower risk of heart disease. They are relaxed, patient, and noncompetitive in their approach to life, experiencing little need for advancement and achievement. This personality is supportive to others and very direct in their approach to situations. They are very social and like to travel and be part of a group. This type is often found in sales, advertising, marketing, public speaking, and party planning and is always willing to work as part of a team.

Type C personalities are cooperative and appealing, unassertive and patient. This type is compliant with authority and not likely to express negative emotions like anger, anxiety, fear, or sadness. They tend to be self-sacrificing, meeting other's needs rather than their own. Breast cancer occurs far more often in women who have a melancholic, rather than sanguine or cheerful temperament. This type of behavior is found in cancer patients.

Yoga

The word yoga, as people in the West understand it, has come down from the biblical word "yoke." The original word, in Sanskrit, is *jugit*. A *yogi* is a person who has learned to relate to the supreme consciousness, which is God. *Yoga* is a union of the individual with the higher consciousness.

Yoga was originally used to maintain a healthy mind in a healthy body, but its continuing and expanding use has led to widespread consideration of yoga as a healing technique. The variety of yoga techniques for breathing and positioning the body are designed to improve both mental and physical well-being and reduce tension by allowing the body to relax. It is an important road to real happiness, tranquility, inner peace, and harmony. Yoga is a form of exercise of mind and body that relieves stress, relaxes us, and prepares us for healing.

Meditation and prayer

Meditation opens a quiet place inside a person that can produce a shift in awareness. When done over time, it is a blessing because more channels of awareness are opened, which creates a basis for growth. Meditation allows you to accomplish many things. Self-improvement also results in an expansion of self-awareness.

Meditation is used for relaxation, creativity, guidance, and to balance your personality. When we go into that quiet place deep within us for fifteen minutes or longer, revelations come to us quite naturally, and we gain fresh insights on how to meet life's situations correctly. Each moment you meditate, inner peace floods your soul.

Prayer is a healing form of meditation. It can work miracles. The healing element in prayer is faith. Recent years show scientific studies on faith and healing. Some of the most important of these have been conducted at Georgetown University School of Medicine in Washington, D.C. Scientists studied patients there who were suffering from pain and crippling rheumatoid arthritis. Although some patients were not present, all were prayed for, even at a distance. Improvement manifested itself the next day in some cases, even though the patients did not know they were being prayed for. Not only did all improve at the end of six months, but also some patients no longer needed medication.

There were also studies done on church goers. People who attend church often have a strong sense of faith, and prayer helps reduce stress. Studies showed that, on the average, those who pray are three times as likely to survive open-heart surgery than those who do not, and they are 70 percent less prone to coronary heart disease. They are also less likely to develop high blood pressure and have a lower rate of depression and anxiety. The studies also showed that people who consider their body the "temple of God," treat it with reverence. Mormons and Seventh-Day Adventists are denominations that lead healthful lifestyles as part of their religious activities. The study also reveals that regular involvement in religious activities can add seven to fourteen years to your life span.

Healing negative emotions

Negative emotions can reduce your happiness and that of people around you. These emotions can cause problems at both a conscious and a subconscious level. They may have their origin in traumatic experiences from your past. Even though the past is history, you may presently still carry some of the emotions with you. You need to learn to heal those emotions. Heal your own anger, guilt, depression, anxiety, envy, fear, phobias, sadness, grief, shame, jealousy, and other unpleasant feelings. Let go of the past completely and learn to live in the present. This healing involves self-honesty, self-acceptance, and the willingness to start living a better life now. Your emotions are your own resources and your own responsibility. No one else can heal your emotions. You, and only you, can do it. Emotional healing is an inside job. You can feel healing take place inside your own body. As negative emotions heal, your life will change for the better.

Anger

We all know what anger is, and we have all felt it. Anger is a completely normal and usually healthy human emotion. When it gets out of control, it can be destructive. It can lead to problems in our personal life. Anger is an emotional state that varies in intensity from mild irritation to intense fury and rage. Physiological changes take place when we get angry. Our heart rate and blood pressure go up, as do the levels of our energy hormones, adrenaline, and noradrenaline. Feelings and behaviors, which allow us to fight and defend ourselves when we are attacked, are necessary to our survival. On the other hand, you can't lash out at every person that irritates or annoys you. It is necessary to learn to moderate anger and to control it—before it controls you.

Anger can be suppressed, but this type of response is dangerous because it turns the anger in on you. Anger turned inward may cause hypertension (high blood pressure) or depression. Even passive-aggressive behavior (i.e., getting back at people indirectly) can turn on you and undermine relationships and health. These people are constantly putting others down, criticizing, and making cynical comments because they haven't learned how to express anger constructively. Such people are not likely to have successful relationships.

Fear

Fear will raise its frightful head any time and any place. Many people have fear of health problems as soon as they hear of someone else with health problems. A persistent irrational fear of an object, activity, or situation is a phobia. Phobias cause panic that is out of proportion to the threat. Common phobias are those involving animals or insects, high places, flying, and many others. These fears are not always considered abnormal. Often, there may be a reason for that fear. Then they are rational fears. They interfere with normal functioning and can be dealt with in a rational way. When we have fear out of proportion to the threat, it may cause symptoms such as anxiety, sweating, poor motor control, rapid heart rate, and a feeling of weakness. Because these are phobias, they cannot be dealt with rationally and may require the help of a therapist.

Guilt

Guilt tells us that we have fallen short of expectations, that we've failed our loved ones and family, that we are selfish to say "no." Guilt is an accuser. Sometimes guilt is a reminder of past mistakes, regrets, and failures. Sometimes it's the threat that others will be hurt or disappointed by our actions. Guilt is slippery and controlling and hard to shake off. Guilt can be beneficial when it reminds us of a past transgression that we have not yet come to terms with. Guilt can be bad when it pressures us into falling in line with unrealistic or even unhealthy human expectations.

Grief

Grief is the normal response of sorrow and confusion that comes from losing someone or something important to us. It is a natural part of life. Grief is a typical reaction to death, divorce, job loss, separation from family and friends, or loss of health. Just after a death or loss, you may feel empty or numb, as if you are in shock. You may notice physical changes such as trembling, nausea, difficulty breathing, muscle weakness, dry mouth, or trouble sleeping and eating. You may become easily angry. Almost everyone in grief experiences guilt. Guilt is often expressed as "I could have," and "I wish I would have." People in grief may have strange dreams or nightmares or become absent-minded and experience social withdrawal. They may lack the desire to return to work.

Time spent grieving is different for each person. There are many reasons for these differences, including personality, health, coping style, culture, family background, and life experiences. It also depends on your relationship with the person lost and how prepared you are for the loss. Try accepting the loss. Work through it and feel the physical and emotional pain of grief. Adjust to living in this world without the person and move on with life. If you are not moving on with your life after a reasonable period of grieving, seek help. It's available.

Develop a positive philosophy

Success can be achieved when a person has a positive outlook on life. Even before undertaking a task, if an individual feels doubtful about the outcome, his whole attitude may prevent achieving success. This does not mean that anyone can attempt any task and achieve success. You must ask, "Am I

equipped to undertake the task at hand?" Sometimes
we know, and again, sometimes we don't know.
However, the power of positive thinking is the key
to getting well.

Some see positive thinking as a cliché. It worked
for me, and I know it will work for you. I have always had the feeling that my higher power was with
me to guide me and keep me safe. I must say, a job
well done! There were times when I felt alone and
did not know what to do, for I had no skills. My main
challenge was making a better living for my daughter
and me. My positive attitude enabled me to come
out successfully. A positive attitude is one which says,
"I will improve what I can, and gracefully accept
what I cannot change."

Autonomy

When my husband passed away, I felt lonely and
did not know what to do. I finally got it together and
realized that I was alone and had a child to care for.
We came to California from Louisiana to live with
my brother and his wife. My dear sister-in-law looked
after my daughter, while I went to work. I did do-
mestic and factory work. When I had saved enough
money, we moved two blocks away from my brother's
house to a one-bedroom apartment. We felt so happy
to have an apartment of our very own. I learned to
drive and bought an old car from my brother. I married, divorced, and went back to school part-time. I
earned a bachelor's degree in child development. We

were very happy. Unfortunately, I married again and later divorced.

Eventually, I was able to buy a house. My daughter and I always felt we had each other. Purchasing a house gave us a base for building a life together. We had nothing but each other. I think my daughter knew what I was trying to do, and what our roles were. We looked forward to the weekends and had good times together. Weekends for me meant sleeping late; for her it meant getting up early to watch cartoons on television. In time, she finished high school and was on her way to college. I was employed in college teaching. We were happier than we had been for a long time. There was still more work to be done. My mother said, "Take care of your own business. If you have time to take care of the other person's business, there is something in your business going undone." I developed this philosophy. It is scary and astonishing to realize that I have been doing things without a great deal of understanding, yet I've made progress. I see this world as a good place to be despite the unrest. We are all born into a system of giving and receiving. Either we take part in it, or we don't; it is the only way we live. We have friends that visit, and we party together, having wonderful times.

I went through a very stressful part of my life balancing work and school, taking care of my daughter, and getting rid of unnecessary, harmful baggage I was carrying. There were many unpleasant experiences along the way. My upbringing helped, along with the joy of my accomplishments.

CHAPTER 10

Spiritual Development and Healing

SPIRIT, THE NEGLECTED ELEMENT IN WESTERN HEALING

I RECOGNIZE THAT SPIRITUAL POWER exists, and that it is always available. I may not know how to access the spiritual solution, but I recognize that it exists and invite the power to be known to me. I feel that the spiritual force is everywhere, in everything, and in everyone. Knowing this, I was determined to forget the concept that some diseases are incurable. What does that say to God? "I give up on You and on myself as an extension of You, as well." Right?

To become whole and healthy, we must balance the body, mind, and spirit. We need to take good care of our bodies, and we need to have a strong spiritual connection. When these three things are balanced, we enjoy living. No doctor or health-care professional can give us this unless we choose to take part in our own healing process.

Traditional Western medicine is mechanistic. Doctors and other health-care specialists picture the body as a machine, with separate parts that must be treated individually. This kind of belief defines the role of the physicians as they treat disease. This way of thinking downplays the mental and emotional factors that may cause or contribute to disease and ignores completely the spiritual aspect of health and well-being.

The body-mind approach to health requires more from you than conventional medicine does. It demands that you educate yourself about the ways your body and mind work together, setting the stage for health or illness. It requires you to exchange bad habits that undermine your health for better habits that promote health. And it dictates that you take responsibility for your health and healing. If a person is depressed, he quite often goes to the doctor and gets an antidepressant and feels better. The pill changes the brain chemistry. Why not learn to think differently, using your own brain? However, learning to think differently takes a lot more work than opening a bottle. If you want to use the body-mind approach to health, you need to do your own research—and that means lots of reading and lots of experimenting. It also requires sorting through all the information, misinformation, good advice, misguided advice, and brilliant insight out there. You need to figure out what works and what does not work through trial and error. This is what I had to do under adverse conditions when I was so ill.

Most of us know about the body-mind connection, but generally, the doctors are still practicing healthcare as usual. Spirituality does not exist for most of them.

I believe we are all spiritual beings. Connecting with the spirit is part of being human. Our bodies are nourished with spiritual energy and guidance. You need to have trust and faith, for they are an important part of creating health. When you have faith in something that is greater then you are, you are in touch with your inner source of power. Each of us has this spark. We just need to go within to find it. We need go no further than ourselves to locate it. Connect with divine guidance. Ask the universe for help to get you there. The guidance will come. Release all expectations of what will happen as a result. Express yourself fully to create health, happiness, and spiritual growth. The way to best express this divine part of yourself is by becoming all of who you truly are. Your body directs you toward full, personal expression by letting you know what feels good and right, and conversely, what does not. Illness is often (but not always) a sign that you are somehow off track.

Spirit, yet to be recognized in mainstream Western medicine

Medical schools should teach the need to address the patient's spiritual or religious concerns to provide better care. Patients express their spiritual views especially when they experience a great deal of pain, when death is near, or if they suffer from chronic illness. Unfortunately, it is the doctor who often does not respond. The doctor may see spirituality as part of counseling and therefore, not part of his profession. There are so many variables as to why the medical and spiritual parts of development are not connected. Some doctors may not feel good about asking open-ended questions. Many physicians may feel only the family physician should get involved in spiritual aspects of the family. This may be an on-going question.

Eastern systems have long recognized the reality of a vital healing force that goes beyond the mind in the healing equation. Eastern thought is concerned about healing the whole person. There are many healing systems, some of which are the martial arts and yoga. They are a part of alternative medicine.

Yoga stresses that awareness, breath, and movement are all part of the healing process. It is often said that awareness is the first step in changing physically, mentally, emotionally, and spiritually. Our body is meant to move and exercise. If our lifestyle does not include opportunities for the natural exercise of muscles and joints, then disease and discomfort will come with time. Proper exercise is pleasant to the body, mind, and spirit. Yoga teaches us how to use the lungs to their maximum capacity and how to control the breath. Proper breathing should be deep, slow, and rhythmical. This increases vitality and mental clarity. Relaxation is of the utmost importance in life. Long before cars, planes, telephones, computers, freeways, and other modern triggers of stress existed, the *Rishis* (sages, seers, and yogis) devised very powerful techniques for deep relaxation.

Many modern stress-management and relaxation methods borrow heavily from yoga. By relaxing all the muscles deeply, the yogi can thoroughly rejuvenate his nervous system and attain a deep sense of inner peace at the same time.

Food plays an important role. Not only does it build a physical body, but also the food we eat profoundly affects our minds. For maximum body-mind efficiency and complete spiritual awareness, yoga advocates a lacto-vegetarian diet—no meat, fish, fowl, animal byproducts (eggs), but some dairy products are allowed. This is an integral part of the yoga lifestyle. But the most important part of all concerns positive and creative thoughts, as these contribute to vibrant health and a peaceful, joyful mind. A positive outlook on life can be acquired. The mind can be brought under perfect control by the regular practice of meditation. In practicing these disciplines, we strive to be healthy. The body, mind, and spirit connection is accomplished through yoga, which is thousands of years old.

Chinese and Japanese martial arts are systems of physical and mental training used for self-understanding, expression through movement, and self-defense. Nowadays, individuals are taking to martial arts as a health practice for life. These disciplines are used to balance the body's organs to relieve pain, cramps, or just relax the body. The most popular martial techniques that have developed in China and Japan are: T'ai Chi Ch'uan (Chinese), Aikido (Japanese), Chi Gung or Qi Gong (Chinese), Judo (Japanese), Jujitsu (Japanese), Karate (Japanese), Kung Fu (Chinese), and Tae Kwon Do (Korean).

Martial arts teach healing techniques and channeling the life force, or *chi*. Training in martial arts can be healthy for the mind, body, and spirit. Done slowly, these arts can build health and cultivate peace of mind. Performed rapidly, the gestures can unleash devastating blows for self-defense. Aikido is based on give-and-take, and is always done with partners. T'ai Chi combines meditation, motion, and deep breathing, increasing the supply of blood, which, in turn, opens blood vessels and allows the heart to function more smoothly. It also opens the joints, especially those of the knees, alleviating inflammatory diseases such as arthritis and rheumatism, and strengthens the lower back. It can improve balance, sharpens memory and concentration, and relieves stress and pain. All of the arts increase psychic energy.

Yoga and all forms of martial arts should not be taken up without consulting your doctor. When you are ready to begin, read some of the many books on styles. However, it is essential to start with a teacher. Movements are too subtle and complex to learn without a coach to encourage and correct the initial efforts. The long-term benefits come from long-term practice. They range from improving muscle tone and physiological self-regulation to cultivating poise and a tranquil spirit. The gentle leg-raising movements massage and strengthen the intestines, aiding in waste elimination. The slow and gentle turning and bending motions massage other organs. Techniques such as T'ai Chi Ch'uan are known to stimulate various acupuncture points.

Alternative healthcare

The philosophy of *chiropractics* is based upon the body's innate intelligence to heal itself. In 1895, Dr.

Daniel David Palmer, the father of chiropractics, gave it its name which means, 'done by hand.' The body seeks to maintain homeostasis and chiropractic manipulations seek to restore it by increasing flexibility and joint functioning, as well as increasing resistance to disease. Chiropractics can also help reduce stress, improve posture, prevent spinal disc degeneration, and improve organ functions. It also relieves pressure on nerves, which chiropractors believe, increases nerve flow. The chiropractor touches the spine to detect vertebral misalignment, or partial dislocation of the vertebrae. When bone has moved out of alignment, there is an interference in the transmission of nerve signals to various organs, resulting in disharmony. The body cannot adapt easily to stresses and healing is impaired. Chiropractics is a natural approach that does not use drugs or surgery. The chiropractor views the body holistically.

Chiropractors believe that when nerves become compressed or stretched, inflammation and irritation occur. Pain results and with the passage of time, there is a decrease in organ function.

Joint damage occurs when there is a locking (fixation) of misaligned vertebral joints, resulting in a decrease in the joints' range of motion. When the spine is misaligned, the discs between vertebrae become compressed over time.

Eventually muscles become weakened and, as a result, tighten and contract. This often causes postural distortions, which affects organ performance.

Misalignment can affect our immune system, causing abnormal hormonal responses and can decrease our adaptation to life's stresses. Disease is the result of inability to adapt to stress. The body loses energy, and degeneration quickly follows. The chiropractor works with the entire spinal column. Spinal check-ups can be as important to your child's health as checkups for eyes, ears, and teeth. These are very good reasons to visit the chiropractor.

Homeopathy is another modern alternative to healthcare, which Dr. Samuel Frederick introduce in 1796. Homeopathy—a highly effective system of medicine developed and practiced since the 18th century—is once again gaining increasing recognition and acceptance as a "modern and natural system of medicine." The vital force, according to homeopathic philosophy, is a dynamic force that flows throughout the body and maintains the normal functioning of mind, body, and soul. *Simile Simibus Curanteur* means that 'the very substance which will produce the symptoms of a disease in a healthy individual can be used to cure a sick person of an illness which causes similar symptoms.' *Homeopathic* means 'to cure by the same pathology.' This therapeutic method consists of giving the patient diluted, but energized, doses of the remedy on the principle of *similia smilibus caranteur*. The method of potentization is a process of progressive dilution with vigorous shaking between each dilution. Based on the principle of *Similia Similibus Curanteur*, when a potentiazed (energized) remedy is introduced into the body of the diseased individual, it energizes the deranged vital force and brings it back to normal.

Homeopathic medicines are safe. They are called remedies to distinguish them from crude drugs usually prescribed and sold at the pharmacy. The amount of the original ingredients in remedies is calculated by the decimal scale and is indicated by a number and the letter "X." The 3X potency contains 1/1,000,000th part of the remedy. The layman should not attempt to take higher potencies except on the advice of a health-care professional. These remedies are nonaddicting and non-habit forming. Homeopathic medicines have been very well accepted recently in countries like the USA, France, Germany, the United Kingdom, Belgium, Italy, Switzerland, and India.

Spirit, a key to healing disease

My father was a Methodist minister. We children had to attend church all day Sunday and had daily prayers in our house. Prayers were said before each meal and before going to bed. My personal agenda in attending church on Sunday was to socialize with my friends and play games. But when I became ill, my spiritual upbringing was there for me. I did not realize it at the time, but it was like an automatic response. I reached for it, and there it was, waiting. Spirituality is a powerful force. I prayed, especially when I was in a lot of pain, and the pain lessened. I would cheer up after being so down. Prayer was one of the rituals that brought me through. The more I learned, the more I used positive thinking in my life. Yoga taught me many things besides breathing and meditation. My nutritionist taught me much about good food. My early religious and spiritual training enhanced the way I conducted myself. I did not panic. I knew healing would be a slow process for me. I had faith that God would do what is right. I attended church regularly and went for daily walks. I began to seek advice from others. I focused each morning on myself. In the evenings, I said to myself, "How can I make tomorrow better?" I believed I could. I had trust in myself and in a higher power. I began to forgive others and myself and moved out of the emotional bag of fear, anger, and guilt. I moved on to a better place in life where there is love, happiness, and peace.

Integrity

What does it mean to have integrity? Is it important to have it? How does having it or not having it impact our lives? Webster defines integrity as 'the quality or state of being unimpaired, of sound moral principles, upright, honest, and sincere.' Having been reared in a home that respected these values, I was conditioned to desire and strive for the best. When you are young, you obey your elders. This includes parents and teachers. By the time you reach adulthood, you are still following rules. I was taught not to make commitments I could not keep. This helped me maintain my sense of honor and dignity, because if I did not keep a commitment, I had an uncomfortable feeling about how I conducted myself. We all know the frustration of being lied to. My upbringing causes me to take issue with it. I learned that we all see things from different perspectives. At home, I learned to be true to my own perspective and to respect those of others.

When learning what it takes to maintain personal integrity, we make mistakes. Doing our best might involve forgiving ourselves for repeating old habits or apologizing to another person. By following these rules, I have been able to make changes for the better over time.

Religious faith

When the sun is not shining, I still know it is there. The key to getting through any challenge is faith. That is, believing what your eyes cannot see. Faith is such a good feeling when you are faced with doubt. Faith is there saying, "I know you believed in me." I am part of faith. Without faith, I could not exist. The love I have for my daughter and believing we can have a better life are feelings that grew out of my faith. I have felt silence in my life. Then I felt I was in a place of horror and darkness. This is when I drew on faith and connected with my spirit as never before. Religious faith helps me and is the foundation of my life. Faith is something that activates me in having confidence to overcome a tragedy, disappointment, loss, or failure, and to bounce back again, looking for and expecting to have a better life.

When I think of faith, I think of President Carter, who said, "One of the most interesting verses I know in the Bible is when the Romans asked Paul what the important things in life were, the things that never changed. Interestingly, Paul answered, 'They're the things that you cannot see.'" What are the things you cannot see that are important? I would suggest justice, truth, humility, service, compassion, and love. You can't see any of those. You can't prove that they're there, but they are guiding lights in a person's life. We need to instill these principles to live by in our lives and our children's lives.

When I began yoga classes, I was introduced to numerous ways to meditate. Meditation helped me to be more aware of myself and my relationship to my surrounding environment and the world in general. When meditating, I feel a growth within my spirit and everything is more meaningful, as if this is what my body needs.

This combination of yoga and meditation helped me to become a better person. I was more creative, more intuitive, and more balanced. As I became more relaxed, my world became more manageable. I learned to meditate in my many yoga poses, sitting in a quiet place, relaxing. Breathing helped me to relax and heal. When I integrated these activities into my daily regimen, I was well on my way to being healed. Later, I became an instructor and chose yoga as the principal exercise I wanted to follow.

It frightens me to think of what would have happened to me if I had continued to be medicated and had put myself through all kinds of expensive tests and needless suffering for the rest of my life. Incorporating a spiritual element in my search was my salvation.

The role of meditation, prayer, and yoga in my healing

Meditation, prayer, and yoga were all part of my healing. You can't have lupus and practice yoga because you hurt all over, and you can't practice yoga and have scleroderma because the skin on the body is too tight. I kept reminding myself that I was healed of lupus and scleroderma. I kept telling Raynaud's disease to go away, but it stayed around part of the time. I think cold hands and feet are more of a psychological problem than the symptoms of the other diseases. When I can keep myself in a relaxed state, Raynaud's goes away. I use biofeedback to keep warm as a backup. I have been consistent, for the most part, under adverse conditions. I know what pain is; there is no way around it. You have to go through it.

Today I am thankful for natural healing. This, I know, very well. I lived through this dark storm. All the methods I used are part of me today; I will never let them go. Since lupus and scleroderma passed through my body, my body knows they were there. I am forever thankful and grateful. I have passed beyond them and today I live a beautiful life.

Conclusion

BY USING MY MIND IN a constructive manner, I changed my behavior, and I became more productive. Because of my illnesses, I had no other choice but to retire from teaching and take care of my health. This gave me time to think, rest, and listen to my body. As I learned useful information and applied it, I began changing little by little, and the stronger I became.

Meditation and prayer started my healing. The support group I joined taught me that *I* needed to find a cure. My family and friends still cannot believe I was seriously ill from auto-immune diseases when they look at me today and see how well I am.

During the years I was very ill, I thought of my past accomplishments and considered the possibility of going back to teaching. I had no idea to do so would take so long. I did manage to teach yoga even while I was ill, because it helped me and aided others.

Writing is something I have always wanted to do. However, I never thought I would be writing and sharing from my own experiences with disease. After

I learned I indeed had scleroderma, lupus, and Raynaud's disease, the medical doctors told me there was no cure for them. I believed their words for a while. This information about "no cure" stayed in my head for a long time. Then one day, I decided not to let this "no cure" business depress me any longer. No more suffering for me. Trial and error, meditation, and prayer led the way for changes. I learned to take charge of my health, and now I am sharing my story, my truth, with you.

Today I feel well. My health has improved beyond my wildest dreams. I walk three miles each morning, five days a week. I practice yoga three times a week. I substitute-teach at a local college. I am productive; I am happy; I am whole. It has taken me fifteen years to find a cure, but my health today is my reward.

References

1. Pauling, Linus. 1986. *How to Live Longer and Feel Better*. New York: Avon Books.

2. Malstrom, Stan D.N.O., MT. 1977. *Own Your Own Body*. New Canaan, CT: Keats Publishing, Inc.

3. Hay, Louise. 1984. *Heal Your Body*. Carlsbab, CA: Hay House, Inc.

4. Conture, Gary L. and Lee Gladden. 1979. *How to Win the Aging Game*. Newport Beach, CA: Habour House Publishers, Inc.

5. Prabhavananda, Swami and Christopher Isherwood. 1981. *How to Know God*. Vedanta Press.

6. Burger, Stuart M. 1988. *How to Be Your Own Nutritionist*. New York: Avon Books.

7. Kellman, Raphael. 2002. *Gut Reaction*. New York: Random House, Inc.

8. Parker, William R. 1957. *Prayer Changes Your Life*. Carmel, New York: Guidepost Associates, Inc.

9. Kloss, Jethro. 1984. *Back to Eden*. Back to Eden Publishing Co.

10. Hefen, Bent Q. and Kathryn J. Frandsen. 1983. *From Acupuncture To Yoga*. Prentice Hall/Hall., Inc., Englewood, New Jersey.

BOOK AVAILABLE THROUGH
Milligan Books, Inc.

Struck Down by Auto–Immune Disease:
How I was Forced to Find My Own Cure - $13.95

Order Form

Milligan Books, Inc.

1425 W. Manchester Ave., Suite C, Los Angeles, CA 90047

(323) 750-3592

Name_____ Date _____

Address _____

City_____ State____ Zip Code ____

Day Telephone _____

Evening Telephone _____

Book Title _____

Number of books ordered___ Total.......... $ _____

Sales Taxes (CA Add 8.25%).................... $ _____

Shipping & Handling $4.90 for one book . $ _____

Add $1.00 for each additional book .... $ _____

Total Amount Due .... $ _____

☐ Check ☐ Money Order ☐ Other Cards _____

☐ Visa   ☐ MasterCard Expiration Date _____

Credit Card No. _____

Driver License No. _____

Make check payable to Milligan Books, Inc.

_____   _____

Signature   Date